CHAPTER 1: INTRODUCTION TO MINIMALLY INVASIVE DENTISTRY

Minimally Invasive Dentistry (MID) represents a paradigm shift in dental practice, emphasizing the preservation of tooth structure and patient comfort. As dentistry has evolved, so too have the techniques and philosophies guiding it. This chapter aims to introduce the core principles of MID, exploring its historical context, fundamental concepts, benefits, and goals. By understanding these aspects, practitioners can better appreciate the shift from traditional invasive methods to modern, patient-centered approaches.

The evolution of MID can be traced back to the growing recognition of the importance of conserving natural tooth structure. Traditional dental practices often involved extensive removal of tooth material to address caries or other dental issues. This approach, while effective in treating the immediate problem, frequently led to the loss of healthy tooth structure and increased susceptibility to future dental issues. As dental science advanced, it became clear that a more conservative approach could offer significant advantages. MID emerged as a response to these concerns, focusing on preserving as much of the natural tooth as possible while still effectively managing dental conditions.

The principles of MID are grounded in a patient-centered philosophy that prioritizes minimal intervention and maximal preservation. The primary goal of MID is to maintain the integrity of healthy tooth structure while addressing dental problems. This involves using advanced diagnostic tools, such as digital imaging and caries detection devices, to identify issues at an early stage. By detecting problems early, dentists can employ less invasive treatment options that require minimal removal of tooth structure. This approach not only enhances the longevity of the treated tooth but also improves overall patient comfort and reduces the likelihood of future complications.

One of the key concepts in MID is the use of preventive measures to avoid the need for more extensive treatment. This involves promoting good oral hygiene practices, regular dental check-ups, and the use of fluoride treatments to strengthen tooth enamel. Preventive care is a cornerstone of MID, as it helps to reduce the incidence of dental problems before they require intervention. By focusing on prevention, dentists can reduce the need for invasive procedures and support the long-term health of their patients' teeth.

Another important aspect of MID is the use of minimally invasive restorative techniques. These techniques aim to repair damaged teeth with the least amount of intervention possible. For example, when treating carious lesions, MID practitioners may use techniques such as air abrasion or laser therapy to remove decay without the need for traditional drilling. These methods not only reduce discomfort for the patient but also preserve more of the healthy tooth structure. Additionally, advancements in dental materials, such as composite resins and glass ionomer cements, have made it possible to restore teeth with highly aesthetic and durable materials that closely mimic natural tooth structure.

The benefits of MID extend beyond the preservation of tooth structure and patient comfort. Minimally invasive techniques can also lead to improved treatment outcomes and reduced treatment times. By avoiding extensive removal of tooth material, the risk of complications such as tooth sensitivity or fracture is minimized. Furthermore, less invasive procedures often require fewer appointments and less time in the dental chair, which can be particularly advantageous for patients with busy schedules or those who experience dental anxiety.

The goals of MID are multifaceted, aiming to enhance both the short-term and long-term outcomes of dental treatment. In the short term, MID seeks to provide effective treatment with minimal discomfort and disruption to the patient's daily life. This involves using advanced techniques and technologies to achieve optimal results while minimizing the impact on the patient. In the long term, MID aims to preserve the natural tooth structure, reduce the need for future dental interventions, and support the overall oral health of the patient.

In conclusion, the introduction to Minimally Invasive Dentistry sets the stage for a deeper understanding of its principles, benefits, and goals. By focusing on the preservation of tooth structure and the use of advanced, patient-centered techniques, MID represents a significant advancement in dental practice. As the field of dentistry continues to evolve, the principles of MID will play an increasingly important role in shaping how dental care is delivered, ensuring that patients receive the highest quality care with the least amount of intervention necessary.

As the field of dentistry progresses, the shift towards minimally invasive techniques reflects broader changes in medical and healthcare practices. Minimally Invasive Dentistry (MID) builds upon a foundation of preventive care and technology-driven approaches to enhance patient outcomes. By emphasizing the preservation of natural tooth structure and reducing intervention whenever possible, MID offers a more patient-centered approach compared to traditional methods.

The philosophical shift towards MID began with a deeper understanding of dental caries and tooth erosion. Historically, treatments for dental caries often involved extensive removal of tooth structure to eliminate decay. While effective, this approach frequently compromised the tooth's long-term health, increasing the risk of future complications such as fractures or additional decay. Modern research has highlighted the importance of preserving as much of the natural tooth as possible, leading to the development of techniques designed to minimize tooth loss while effectively managing carious lesions.

MID's emphasis on preservation involves using advanced diagnostic tools to detect dental issues at their earliest stages. Techniques such as digital radiography, fiber-optic transillumination, and laser fluorescence provide detailed insights into tooth structure and the extent of decay. These tools allow for more accurate diagnosis and enable practitioners to select the most appropriate and least invasive treatment options. For example, digital imaging can identify early carious lesions that might be missed with traditional methods, allowing for interventions that target only the affected areas without unnecessary removal of healthy tissue.

The development of advanced materials has also played a crucial role in the rise of MID. Innovations in dental materials have enabled practitioners to restore teeth with greater precision and durability while preserving natural tooth structure. Composite resins, for instance, are used to fill cavities with materials that closely mimic the appearance and function of natural tooth enamel. These materials can be applied with minimal preparation of the tooth structure, thus reducing the invasiveness of the procedure. Similarly, glass ionomer cements release fluoride, which helps in the prevention of further decay, supporting the MID philosophy of preventive care.

Restorative techniques in MID focus on minimally invasive methods that are designed to preserve healthy tooth structure while repairing damage. Air abrasion and laser therapy are examples of such techniques. Air abrasion uses a stream of fine particles to remove decayed tissue without the need for traditional drills. This method not only reduces discomfort but also allows for more precise removal of affected areas. Laser therapy, on the other hand, uses concentrated light to remove decayed tissue and can also be used for procedures like tooth whitening and soft tissue surgery. Both of these methods align with the principles of MID by minimizing the impact on surrounding healthy tissues.

Furthermore, MID emphasizes the integration of preventive strategies into routine dental care. Preventive measures, such as regular fluoride treatments, dental sealants, and patient education on proper oral hygiene, are integral to reducing the need for invasive treatments. Fluoride treatments strengthen tooth enamel, making it more resistant to decay, while dental sealants provide a protective barrier against caries, particularly in the pits and fissures of molars. By focusing on prevention, MID aims to reduce the incidence of dental problems before they require more extensive intervention.

Patient comfort is a key consideration in MID. Traditional dental procedures can often be associated with discomfort and anxiety, which can deter patients from seeking necessary care. Minimally invasive techniques, by reducing the extent of intervention, contribute to a more comfortable experience for the patient. Additionally, advancements in local anesthesia and sedation options further enhance patient comfort, making dental procedures less daunting and more accessible.

The benefits of MID extend beyond immediate patient comfort and treatment outcomes. By preserving natural tooth structure and reducing the need for extensive interventions, MID contributes to the long-term health and stability of dental restorations. Teeth treated with minimally invasive techniques are less likely to experience complications such as fractures or recurrent decay, leading to better overall outcomes and reduced need for future treatments.

As the field of MID continues to evolve, ongoing research and technological advancements will likely bring about further innovations. The integration of digital technologies, such as artificial intelligence and machine learning, may enhance diagnostic accuracy and treatment planning. These technologies hold the potential to further refine minimally invasive techniques and improve patient outcomes.

In summary, Minimally Invasive Dentistry represents a significant advancement in dental care, focusing on the preservation of natural tooth structure and minimizing patient discomfort. By leveraging advanced diagnostic tools, materials, and techniques, MID offers a more conservative and patient-centered approach to dental treatment. As dental practices continue to embrace these principles, the field of MID will play a pivotal role in shaping the future of oral healthcare, promoting long-term tooth health and patient well-being.

As the field of dentistry advances, the principles of Minimally Invasive Dentistry (MID) continue to gain traction, driven by an increasing emphasis on patient-centered care and technological innovation. The integration of MID into everyday practice reflects a broader commitment to enhancing both the effectiveness of dental treatments and the overall patient experience.

One of the fundamental aspects of MID is its approach to caries management. Traditionally, dental caries were treated by removing all decayed tissue, often resulting in the removal of healthy tooth structure as well. The MID approach, however, focuses on the selective removal of only the diseased tissue, preserving as much of the natural tooth as possible. This is achieved through advanced diagnostic tools and techniques that allow for the precise identification and treatment of carious lesions. For instance, techniques such as laser fluorescence and fiber-optic transillumination offer detailed insights into the extent of decay, facilitating targeted interventions that minimize the impact on healthy tooth structure.

The use of conservative restorative materials is another cornerstone of MID. Modern materials like composite resins and glass ionomer cements not only provide durable and aesthetically pleasing results but also allow for less invasive application. Composite resins, in particular, can be bonded directly to the tooth structure, reducing the need for extensive preparation. Glass ionomer cements, which release fluoride, contribute to the ongoing protection of the tooth and help to prevent future decay. These materials support the MID philosophy by enabling repairs and restorations that align with the principles of minimal intervention.

A significant benefit of MID is its potential to enhance patient comfort and reduce anxiety associated with dental procedures. Traditional invasive treatments often involve drilling and other techniques that can be uncomfortable or intimidating for patients. In contrast, minimally invasive procedures tend to be less traumatic, which can lead to a more positive experience and encourage patients to seek care when needed. For example, techniques such as air abrasion or laser treatment can be performed with minimal discomfort and often require less anesthetic, further contributing to a more pleasant experience.

Patient education and involvement are integral components of

MID. Educating patients about the importance of preventive care, the benefits of minimally invasive techniques, and proper oral hygiene practices empowers them to take an active role in their dental health. MID emphasizes the prevention of dental issues before they require intervention, and this proactive approach aligns with the broader goal of maintaining optimal oral health. By engaging patients in their care and providing them with the tools and knowledge to prevent dental problems, MID fosters a collaborative relationship between the dentist and patient.

The implementation of MID also involves a critical evaluation of existing practices and a willingness to adapt to new methodologies. Dentists must remain informed about advancements in technology and materials to effectively incorporate minimally invasive techniques into their practice. This requires ongoing education and training, as well as a commitment to evaluating the effectiveness of new approaches. The dynamic nature of MID necessitates that dental professionals stay current with emerging trends and research to ensure they are providing the best possible care to their patients.

Looking forward, the future of MID is likely to be shaped by continued advancements in technology and a deeper understanding of dental disease mechanisms. Innovations such as digital imaging, artificial intelligence, and biomaterials are poised to further enhance the precision and efficacy of minimally invasive techniques. For instance, digital imaging technologies may enable even more accurate diagnostics and treatment planning, while advancements in biomaterials could lead to the development of new materials that offer improved durability and functionality.

In summary, Minimally Invasive Dentistry represents a transformative approach to dental care, characterized by its focus on preserving natural tooth structure, minimizing patient discomfort, and emphasizing preventive measures. The evolution of MID reflects a broader trend towards patient-centered care and technological innovation, highlighting the importance of maintaining a conservative approach while effectively addressing dental issues. As the field continues to advance, MID will play an increasingly vital role in shaping the future of dental practice, ensuring that patients receive care that is both effective and aligned with the principles of minimal intervention.

CHAPTER 2: THE PRINCIPLES OF MINIMALLY INVASIVE DENTISTRY

At the heart of Minimally Invasive Dentistry (MID) lies a set of guiding principles that seek to reshape traditional dental practices into more conservative and patient-centered approaches. These principles emphasize the preservation of natural tooth structure, early diagnosis, and preventive care, all of which are integral to the philosophy of MID. Understanding these core concepts provides a foundation for implementing effective and modern dental treatments that align with the ethos of minimal intervention.

Early diagnosis is a cornerstone of MID, reflecting a shift from reactive to proactive dental care. The early identification of dental issues enables practitioners to address problems before they escalate, thus preserving the integrity of the tooth structure and minimizing the need for more invasive procedures. Techniques such as digital radiography and advanced diagnostic tools like laser fluorescence play a crucial role in this aspect. Digital radiography offers high-resolution images with reduced radiation exposure, allowing for the precise detection of carious lesions and other dental anomalies. Laser fluorescence, on the other hand, aids in identifying early-stage carious lesions that might not be visible through conventional imaging methods. By leveraging these technologies, dentists can diagnose dental issues at their inception, facilitating timely and less invasive treatments.

Preventive care is another fundamental principle of MID. This approach focuses on maintaining oral health and preventing the onset of dental issues rather than merely reacting to them. Preventive strategies encompass a range of practices including patient education, routine cleanings, fluoride treatments, and sealants. Educating patients about proper oral hygiene and the importance of regular dental visits empowers them to take an active role in their dental health. Routine cleanings and fluoride treatments help to fortify tooth enamel and prevent decay, while sealants provide an additional layer of protection against carious lesions, particularly in the pits and fissures of molars. Preventive care, therefore, not only helps in averting dental problems but also aligns with the MID philosophy by reducing the need for more invasive interventions in the future.

The preservation of natural tooth structure is a pivotal aspect of MID and reflects its core philosophy. Traditional dental practices often involved extensive removal of tooth material to address decay or damage, which could compromise the long-term health and function of the tooth. In contrast, MID prioritizes the conservation of as much natural tooth structure as possible. This principle is guided by the belief that maintaining the integrity of the tooth is crucial for both its functional longevity and its aesthetic appearance. Modern restorative materials and techniques support this approach by allowing for more precise and conservative interventions. For example, composite resins and glass ionomer cements enable direct bonding to the tooth structure, reducing the need for extensive preparation and preserving the surrounding healthy enamel.

In practice, these principles guide treatment planning and decision-making processes, shaping the way dental professionals approach patient care. When devising a treatment plan, practitioners adhere to the principles of MID by evaluating the least invasive options first and considering the long-term outcomes of various interventions. This involves a careful assessment of the patient's oral health status, including the extent of any existing issues and the potential for future problems. By prioritizing conservative treatments and focusing on preservation and prevention, dentists can enhance the overall quality of care while minimizing patient discomfort and treatment-related anxiety.

The principles of MID also extend to the patient experience, highlighting the importance of a collaborative approach to dental care. Engaging patients in their treatment planning process not only improves adherence to recommended care but also fosters a sense of empowerment and involvement. This collaborative approach is integral to the MID philosophy, as it aligns with the broader goal of creating a patient-centered care environment. By discussing treatment options, explaining the rationale behind minimally invasive approaches, and addressing patient concerns, dentists can build trust and encourage active participation in maintaining oral health.

In summary, the principles of Minimally Invasive Dentistry—early diagnosis, preventive care, and preservation of natural tooth structure—form the foundation of a modern approach to dental practice. These principles reflect a shift towards more conservative and patient-focused care, emphasizing the importance of proactive measures and less invasive interventions. By integrating these principles into treatment planning and patient interactions, dental professionals can enhance the effectiveness and patient satisfaction of their practices while aligning with the overarching goals of MID.

In addition to early diagnosis, preventive care, and preservation of natural tooth structure, Minimally Invasive Dentistry (MID) encompasses several other principles that collectively contribute to its holistic approach. These include the use of advanced materials and techniques, the emphasis on patient-centered care, and the integration of technology in treatment planning and execution.

The application of advanced materials and techniques is integral to the practice of MID. Innovations in dental materials have significantly enhanced the ability to perform less invasive procedures while achieving optimal outcomes. For example, the development of high-strength, tooth-colored materials such as resin composites and ceramics allows for the repair of teeth with minimal removal of healthy tooth structure. These materials not only offer aesthetic advantages but also contribute to the durability and functionality of restorations. Moreover, techniques such as air abrasion and laser dentistry have revolutionized the treatment of carious lesions and other dental conditions. Air abrasion, which uses a stream of fine particles to remove decay, is less invasive than traditional drilling methods and can be employed with greater precision. Laser dentistry, similarly, enables targeted treatment with minimal impact on surrounding tissues, reducing the need for more extensive interventions.

Patient-centered care is a cornerstone of MID and reflects a commitment to addressing individual patient needs and preferences. This approach involves engaging patients in the decision-making process and considering their values and concerns when planning treatments. By fostering open communication and providing clear explanations of treatment options, dental professionals can ensure that patients are well-informed and actively involved in their care. This collaborative approach not only enhances patient satisfaction but also aligns with the principles of MID by promoting treatments that are tailored to each patient's specific needs and conditions.

The integration of technology into dental practice further supports the principles of MID by enhancing diagnostic accuracy and treatment effectiveness. Digital technologies, including intraoral cameras, cone-beam computed tomography (CBCT), and CAD/CAM systems, have transformed how dental professionals assess and treat patients. Intraoral cameras provide detailed images of the oral cavity, allowing for more accurate diagnosis and better patient education. CBCT imaging offers three-dimensional views of dental structures, facilitating precise treatment planning and the evaluation of complex cases. CAD/CAM systems enable the design and fabrication of restorations with high precision, often in a single visit, reducing the need for multiple appointments and interim restorations. These technological advancements not only support the principles of early diagnosis and preservation of tooth structure but also contribute to the overall efficiency and effectiveness of dental treatments.

Another important aspect of MID is the focus on holistic care, which involves considering the overall health and well-being of the patient in addition to their dental needs. This principle acknowledges the interplay between oral health and general health, recognizing that dental conditions can have broader implications for a patient's overall health. For instance, conditions such as periodontal disease have been linked to systemic health issues, including cardiovascular disease and diabetes. By addressing dental problems in a manner that considers their potential impact on overall health, dental professionals can provide more comprehensive care and contribute to the patient's long-term well-being.

Moreover, the philosophy of MID emphasizes the importance of continuous education and professional development for dental practitioners. As advancements in dental science and technology continue to evolve, staying informed about the latest research, techniques, and materials is essential for maintaining high standards of care. Ongoing education enables dental professionals to incorporate new knowledge and practices into their work, ensuring that they can offer the most current and effective treatments to their patients.

In summary, the principles of Minimally Invasive Dentistry extend beyond early diagnosis, preventive care, and preservation of natural tooth structure. They include the use of advanced materials and techniques, a commitment to patient-centered care, the integration of cutting-edge technology, a focus on holistic care, and the importance of continuous professional development. These principles collectively define a modern approach to dental practice that prioritizes conservative and patient-focused treatments, ultimately leading to improved outcomes and enhanced patient satisfaction.

The application of minimally invasive dentistry (MID) principles in clinical practice necessitates a nuanced approach to treatment planning and execution. Each principle—early diagnosis, preventive care, and preservation of natural tooth structure—intersects with various aspects of patient care and clinical decision-making. Understanding how these principles guide and enhance dental practice can help practitioners deliver optimal outcomes while adhering to the MID philosophy.

Early diagnosis is not merely about detecting issues at their nascent stages but also about utilizing advanced diagnostic tools to foresee potential problems before they escalate. The early identification of dental conditions relies heavily on the integration of comprehensive diagnostic technologies. For instance, digital radiography provides high-resolution images that can reveal subtler signs of decay or pathology that might not be visible through traditional methods. The use of fiber-optic transillumination, a technique that highlights carious lesions and cracks by shining light through the tooth, further augments diagnostic capabilities. These technologies enable dentists to recognize and address issues before they require more invasive interventions, thereby aligning with MID principles.

Preventive care extends beyond routine cleanings and check-ups; it encompasses a proactive approach to maintaining oral health through patient education, lifestyle modifications, and targeted preventive treatments. Patient education plays a pivotal role, as it empowers individuals to take responsibility for their oral health through informed decisions about diet, oral hygiene practices, and regular dental visits. For instance, fluoride treatments and sealants are preventive measures that protect teeth from decay and abrasion. These treatments, when used judiciously, not only avert the need for restorative procedures but also reflect the essence of MID by safeguarding the natural tooth structure.

Moreover, preventive care includes the management of risk factors associated with oral diseases. Understanding the patient's overall health, including their medical history and lifestyle choices, allows for a tailored preventive strategy. For example, patients with a history of high caries risk may benefit from more frequent fluoride applications and dietary counseling to reduce their sugar intake. This individualized approach aligns with the principle of preserving tooth structure by mitigating risks before they necessitate more invasive treatments.

The preservation of natural tooth structure is a fundamental tenet of MID, which emphasizes the importance of conserving as much of the tooth as possible while still achieving therapeutic goals. This principle manifests in various treatment strategies, such as conservative cavity preparations, the use of minimally invasive restorative materials, and the application of techniques that limit tooth destruction. For example, when treating carious lesions, the use of atraumatic restorative treatment (ART) techniques can remove decay with minimal impact on healthy tooth structure. Similarly, the application of bonded restorations and resin-based composites helps to restore teeth while maintaining their integrity and function.

In addition to these specific practices, the preservation principle involves a broader understanding of how dental interventions affect long-term tooth health. For instance, the choice between indirect restorations, such as crowns, versus direct restorations, like fillings, can impact the remaining tooth structure. While crowns might offer more extensive coverage, they often require significant tooth reduction. In contrast, fillings, when applied conservatively, help preserve more of the natural tooth. Thus, treatment planning in MID requires a careful balance between addressing immediate dental issues and maintaining the structural integrity of the tooth over time.

Treatment planning guided by MID principles also incorporates a multidisciplinary approach, where necessary. Collaboration with other dental specialists, such as periodontists or orthodontists, can provide a comprehensive care plan that addresses complex cases involving multiple aspects of oral health. For example, an interdisciplinary approach may be required when dealing with severe periodontal disease that affects tooth stability or when planning orthodontic treatment that impacts the alignment and function of teeth. By integrating different specialties, dentists can develop a more holistic treatment strategy that aligns with MID principles.

Finally, the implementation of MID principles in clinical practice is supported by ongoing research and advancements in dental science. As new techniques, materials, and technologies emerge, they offer opportunities to enhance the effectiveness and scope of minimally invasive approaches. Staying abreast of these developments through continuous education and professional development ensures that dental practitioners can apply the most current and effective practices in their work.

In summary, the principles of minimally invasive dentistry—early diagnosis, preventive care, and preservation of natural tooth structure—serve as foundational elements that guide modern dental practice. By integrating advanced diagnostic technologies, adopting proactive preventive measures, and employing conservative treatment strategies, dental professionals can align their practices with the core tenets of MID. These principles not only facilitate effective patient care but also contribute to the advancement of dental science and the overall improvement of oral health outcomes.

CHAPTER 3: DIAGNOSTIC TECHNOLOGIES IN MINIMALLY INVASIVE DENTISTRY

The efficacy of minimally invasive dentistry (MID) relies significantly on the precision of diagnostic technologies used to identify and manage dental issues with minimal intervention. Advanced diagnostic tools are integral to detecting dental conditions at their earliest stages, thereby allowing for timely and less invasive treatments. This chapter delves into the pivotal diagnostic technologies that underpin MID, focusing on advanced imaging techniques such as digital radiography and intraoral cameras, and their role in accurate diagnosis and treatment planning.

Digital radiography represents a significant advancement over traditional film-based radiography, offering enhanced diagnostic capabilities with reduced radiation exposure. Unlike conventional X-rays, which require the development of film and manual processing, digital radiography utilizes electronic sensors to capture and immediately display detailed images on a computer screen. This immediacy not only streamlines the workflow but also allows for greater diagnostic precision. The ability to adjust image contrast and magnify areas of interest further enhances the detection of early-stage dental issues, such as incipient carious lesions or microfractures, which might be missed with conventional radiographic methods.

Another key advantage of digital radiography is its contribution to patient safety and comfort. The lower radiation dose associated with digital sensors minimizes the risk to patients, making it a preferable option for frequent imaging or for vulnerable populations such as children. Additionally, digital images can be easily stored and shared, facilitating better communication between dental professionals and enabling more comprehensive treatment planning.

Intraoral cameras represent another vital tool in the arsenal of minimally invasive diagnostic technologies. These small, hand-held devices are designed to capture high-resolution images and videos of the oral cavity, including areas that are difficult to view directly. The use of intraoral cameras allows for the visualization of the tooth surfaces, gingiva, and restorations in great detail. This capability is instrumental in identifying conditions such as plaque accumulation, early signs of caries, or defective restorations. By providing real-time, magnified images, intraoral cameras assist clinicians in making accurate diagnoses and in educating patients about their oral health conditions.

The integration of intraoral cameras into practice also enhances patient engagement. Visual evidence of dental issues can be shown to patients, fostering a clearer understanding of their condition and the need for specific treatments. This visual feedback can be particularly effective in reinforcing the importance of preventive care and adherence to recommended treatment plans. Moreover, intraoral cameras facilitate better documentation of the patient's oral health over time, which is invaluable for tracking the progression of conditions and evaluating the effectiveness of interventions.

Advanced imaging techniques, such as cone-beam computed tomography (CBCT), further expand the diagnostic capabilities within minimally invasive dentistry. CBCT provides three-dimensional images of the dental structures, including the bones, teeth, and surrounding soft tissues. Unlike traditional two-dimensional radiographs, which can sometimes obscure critical anatomical details, CBCT offers comprehensive views that aid in precise diagnosis and treatment planning. This is particularly useful in complex cases involving implant placement, root canal therapy, and the assessment of jawbone structure. The detailed visualization provided by CBCT allows for more accurate planning and execution of procedures, thereby reducing the need for exploratory surgeries and enhancing the overall efficacy of treatments.

The role of diagnostic technologies in minimally invasive dentistry extends beyond mere detection; they also play a crucial role in monitoring the effectiveness of treatments. For example, after the placement of a conservative restoration or preventive treatment, follow-up imaging can be used to evaluate the success of the intervention and ensure that the condition has been effectively managed. This ongoing assessment helps in maintaining the integrity of the tooth structure and in making any necessary adjustments to the treatment plan.

The continuous evolution of diagnostic technologies presents opportunities for further advancements in MID. Innovations such as artificial intelligence (AI) and machine learning are beginning to play a role in enhancing diagnostic accuracy. AI algorithms can analyze vast amounts of imaging data to identify patterns and anomalies that might be missed by human eyes, thus aiding in the early detection of dental conditions. As these technologies become more refined and integrated into practice, they hold the potential to further improve the precision and effectiveness of minimally invasive approaches.

In conclusion, the role of diagnostic technologies in minimally invasive dentistry is central to the practice's emphasis on early detection and conservative treatment. Digital radiography, intraoral cameras, and advanced imaging techniques like CBCT each contribute to a more detailed and accurate understanding of dental conditions, facilitating timely and less invasive interventions. These tools not only enhance diagnostic capabilities but also improve patient communication and care. As technology continues to advance, the integration of new diagnostic tools will further enhance the practice of minimally invasive dentistry, offering even greater potential for preserving natural tooth structure and improving overall patient outcomes.

The impact of diagnostic technologies in minimally invasive dentistry (MID) extends significantly beyond their mere functionality; these tools shape the fundamental approach to patient care by enabling early detection and facilitating targeted interventions. Understanding how these technologies contribute to a more refined diagnostic process is crucial for appreciating their role in advancing MID practices.

Digital radiography has revolutionized dental imaging with its ability to provide immediate and high-quality images while reducing radiation exposure compared to traditional film-based methods. This technology employs electronic sensors that capture X-ray images, which are then processed and displayed on a computer screen. The immediate availability of these images allows for swift diagnosis and decision-making. Clinicians can easily adjust the image's contrast, brightness, and zoom levels, which enhances the visibility of dental structures and potential anomalies. This capability is particularly beneficial for detecting subtle signs of decay or early-stage carious lesions that might otherwise remain unnoticed.

Moreover, digital radiography integrates seamlessly with modern dental practice management systems, facilitating easier storage, retrieval, and sharing of patient images. This digital integration not only streamlines workflow but also enhances collaborative care. Dentists can share diagnostic images with specialists or refer patients for further evaluation with greater efficiency, supporting a cohesive treatment strategy. The ability to track changes over time through a digital archive of images also aids in monitoring the progression of dental conditions and evaluating the effectiveness of interventions.

Intraoral cameras offer a complementary diagnostic approach by providing direct visualization of the oral cavity. These small, handheld devices are equipped with high-resolution cameras that capture detailed images of the teeth, gums, and other oral tissues. Intraoral cameras allow for real-time visualization and immediate feedback, which is instrumental in identifying conditions such as plaque buildup, early carious lesions, and wear patterns. The magnified images captured by these cameras reveal intricate details that are not always visible with the naked eye or traditional radiographs.

The application of intraoral cameras extends beyond diagnostics to enhance patient education and engagement. By displaying real-time images on a screen, clinicians can effectively communicate the status of a patient's oral health and explain the necessity of recommended treatments. This visual evidence helps patients understand their condition and the rationale behind specific interventions, fostering informed consent and encouraging adherence to treatment plans.

The role of advanced imaging techniques, such as cone-beam computed tomography (CBCT), cannot be overstated in the context of minimally invasive dentistry. CBCT provides three-dimensional images of the dental and maxillofacial structures, offering a comprehensive view that surpasses the capabilities of traditional two-dimensional radiographs. This detailed visualization is particularly valuable for complex diagnostic scenarios, including the planning of implant placements, root canal treatments, and the evaluation of bone structures.

CBCT's three-dimensional imaging allows for precise assessment of anatomical details, which is crucial for planning and executing intricate procedures. For example, in implant dentistry, CBCT enables clinicians to assess bone density, structure, and spatial relationships with high accuracy, thereby improving the placement and stability of dental implants. Additionally, the ability to visualize the relationship between anatomical structures helps in avoiding critical structures, such as nerves and sinuses, reducing the risk of complications during treatment.

Beyond their diagnostic applications, the advanced imaging technologies discussed play a significant role in the ongoing management of dental conditions. The ability to conduct follow-up imaging allows for the evaluation of treatment outcomes and the monitoring of disease progression or resolution. This dynamic approach to patient care aligns with the principles of minimally invasive dentistry by ensuring that treatments are effective and that any necessary adjustments are made promptly.

In addition to these imaging technologies, emerging advancements in artificial intelligence (AI) and machine learning are beginning to transform the diagnostic landscape in dentistry. AI algorithms, trained on vast datasets of dental images, can assist in identifying patterns and anomalies with remarkable precision. These technologies have the potential to enhance diagnostic accuracy, particularly in detecting subtle changes or rare conditions that may be challenging to recognize through conventional means.

The integration of AI into diagnostic processes holds promise for further elevating the standards of care in minimally invasive dentistry. As these technologies evolve, they will likely become increasingly adept at supporting clinicians in making more informed and accurate diagnoses, thereby reinforcing the practice's commitment to preserving tooth structure and minimizing invasive procedures.

In summary, diagnostic technologies in minimally invasive dentistry are pivotal in shaping modern dental practices. Digital radiography and intraoral cameras offer enhanced diagnostic capabilities and improve patient communication, while advanced imaging techniques like CBCT provide comprehensive views essential for complex treatments. The continued development and integration of AI and machine learning technologies promise to further refine diagnostic accuracy and elevate patient care. By leveraging these advanced tools, dental professionals can more effectively implement minimally invasive approaches, ultimately contributing to improved outcomes and enhanced patient experiences.

As diagnostic technologies advance, their integration into minimally invasive dentistry continues to refine the approach to patient care, aligning with the core tenets of early detection and preservation. Understanding these technologies in the context of their applications, benefits, and limitations provides a comprehensive view of their role in modern dental practices.

The use of digital radiography has become a cornerstone in contemporary diagnostic approaches. This technology, by providing immediate feedback and high-resolution images with reduced radiation, allows for an enhanced diagnostic process. Traditional film-based radiography, with its extended development time and higher radiation dose, has largely been supplanted by digital methods that offer a more patient-friendly alternative. Digital radiographs are not only quicker to obtain but also facilitate more precise image manipulation, enabling practitioners to discern finer details of dental structures and detect early signs of carious lesions or structural changes.

A key benefit of digital radiography is its capacity for integration with electronic health records and practice management systems. This digital synergy supports a streamlined workflow, enabling easy access to past and present images, which is invaluable for monitoring the progression of dental issues and assessing the effectiveness of ongoing treatments. Moreover, the ability to enhance and adjust images in real time supports a more accurate diagnosis and facilitates clearer communication with patients regarding their oral health status.

Intraoral cameras serve as another vital tool in the diagnostic arsenal, offering a direct, real-time view of the oral cavity. Their small size and maneuverability allow for detailed examination of areas that may be difficult to access or visualize with other methods. By capturing high-resolution images of the teeth and soft tissues, intraoral cameras provide valuable insights into conditions such as plaque accumulation, gingival inflammation, and initial carious lesions. The immediate feedback offered by these cameras supports a more responsive diagnostic process, enabling clinicians to make well-informed decisions during the patient consultation.

Intraoral cameras also play a crucial role in patient education. By displaying real-time images on a monitor, patients can visually understand the state of their oral health, which enhances their engagement in the diagnostic and treatment planning process. This visual evidence helps in explaining the necessity of specific interventions and reinforces the importance of adherence to preventive care recommendations. Such interactive communication fosters a more collaborative approach to dental care, where patients are more informed and involved in their treatment decisions.

The advent of cone-beam computed tomography (CBCT) represents a significant advancement in imaging technology, providing three-dimensional views of dental and maxillofacial structures. CBCT scans deliver a level of detail and spatial accuracy that two-dimensional radiographs cannot achieve, making it an indispensable tool for complex cases. This technology allows for precise evaluation of bone structure, which is essential for planning procedures such as dental implants, orthognathic surgery, and the assessment of anatomical relationships that could impact treatment outcomes.

CBCT's detailed imaging capabilities extend to its utility in diagnosing conditions that require comprehensive anatomical understanding. For instance, the visualization of the mandibular canal, maxillary sinus, and surrounding bone structures supports the accurate placement of implants, reducing the risk of complications and improving procedural success. Furthermore, CBCT enables the assessment of root canal anatomy and the identification of anatomical variations, which is critical for endodontic treatments.

As the field of minimally invasive dentistry progresses, emerging technologies such as artificial intelligence (AI) and machine learning are beginning to make their mark. AI algorithms, trained on extensive datasets of dental images, are being developed to assist in the diagnostic process by identifying patterns and anomalies with high accuracy. These technologies hold promise for augmenting human expertise by providing additional layers of analysis and supporting more precise diagnostic decisions.

AI's potential in dentistry includes enhanced image analysis, early detection of conditions, and predictive analytics for treatment planning. For example, AI can help in detecting early carious lesions or analyzing changes in dental structures over time, offering insights that might be missed by the human eye. As these technologies evolve, they are likely to become integral components of the diagnostic toolkit, further advancing the principles of minimally invasive care by promoting early intervention and preserving tooth structure.

Despite the advancements, it is essential to acknowledge the limitations and challenges associated with these technologies. For instance, while digital radiography and intraoral cameras offer significant benefits, they also require proper calibration, regular maintenance, and skilled interpretation to ensure accurate diagnostics. Similarly, the high cost of advanced imaging technologies like CBCT may be a barrier for some practices, potentially impacting their accessibility and integration.

In summary, diagnostic technologies in minimally invasive dentistry represent a significant leap forward in enhancing the precision and effectiveness of dental care. Digital radiography, intraoral cameras, and CBCT each offer unique advantages that contribute to early detection, accurate diagnosis, and improved patient outcomes. As these technologies continue to evolve and integrate with emerging advancements such as AI, they will further refine the practice of minimally invasive dentistry, supporting the overarching goals of preserving natural tooth structure and minimizing patient discomfort. Embracing and understanding these technologies is crucial for dental professionals committed to advancing patient care and staying at the forefront of dental practice innovation.

CHAPTER 4: ADHESIVE DENTISTRY AND BONDING TECHNIQUES

Adhesive dentistry has revolutionized the field of restorative dentistry by emphasizing techniques that prioritize the preservation of natural tooth structure while achieving strong, durable restorations. This chapter delves into the complexities of adhesive dentistry, exploring various bonding techniques, types of dental adhesives, and their applications. The principles underlying the bonding process to enamel and dentin are crucial for understanding how these techniques enhance the effectiveness of minimally invasive treatments.

At the heart of adhesive dentistry is the concept of bonding, which involves the application of adhesives to create a strong, lasting connection between restorative materials and the natural tooth structure. This connection is pivotal in ensuring the longevity and functionality of restorations such as fillings, crowns, and veneers. The evolution of bonding techniques has been driven by advances in material science and a deeper understanding of dental hard tissues, enabling more conservative approaches to dental restoration.

The foundation of adhesive dentistry lies in the development of dental adhesives, which are categorized into various types based on their composition and bonding mechanisms. These adhesives generally fall into two main categories: etch-and-rinse adhesives and self-etch adhesives. Each category employs distinct methods to prepare the tooth surface and achieve bonding.

Etch-and-rinse adhesives, also known as total-etch systems, involve a multi-step process that starts with the application of an acidic etchant to the tooth surface. This etching removes the outer layer of enamel or dentin, creating a roughened surface that enhances the adhesive's ability to penetrate and bond. After etching, a primer is applied to further prepare the surface and improve the adhesive's penetration into the dentinal tubules. Finally, a bonding resin is applied, which forms a strong bond with the tooth structure once it is cured with a light source. This technique is well-established and provides reliable results, though it requires meticulous execution of each step to avoid potential issues such as over-etching or inadequate bonding.

Self-etch adhesives, on the other hand, simplify the bonding process by combining the etching and priming steps into a single application. These adhesives contain acidic components that simultaneously etch and prime the tooth surface, eliminating the need for separate steps. This approach reduces the potential for technique errors and offers a more streamlined workflow. Self-etch adhesives are particularly advantageous in situations where a more conservative approach is desired, as they typically result in less enamel loss compared to etch-and-rinse systems. However, they may be less effective in cases where significant dentin bonding is required, as their acidic components may not penetrate as deeply as in total-etch systems.

In addition to etch-and-rinse and self-etch adhesives, there are also universal adhesives that offer versatility in application. Universal adhesives can be used in both etch-and-rinse and self-etch modes, allowing practitioners to adapt their approach based on clinical needs. These adhesives often include advanced formulations that improve adhesion to a variety of substrates, including both enamel and dentin, as well as restorative materials such as composites and ceramics. The flexibility of universal adhesives makes them a valuable tool in modern adhesive dentistry, enabling a more adaptable approach to different clinical scenarios.

Bonding to enamel and dentin involves different considerations due to the distinct properties of these tissues. Enamel, being a highly mineralized and relatively non-porous tissue, bonds well with adhesive systems when properly etched. The etching process removes the organic layer and exposes the enamel rods, creating a surface that readily accepts adhesive resins. In contrast, dentin is more complex due to its organic matrix and presence of dentinal tubules. The bonding process to dentin requires careful management to ensure optimal adhesion without causing excessive moisture interference or collapse of the dentinal collagen network.

The principles of bonding to dentin involve the creation of a hybrid layer, which is formed by the infiltration of adhesive resins into the demineralized dentin. This hybrid layer establishes a strong bond between the dentin and the restorative material by mechanically interlocking with the tooth structure and chemically bonding to the collagen fibers. Successful bonding to dentin is influenced by factors such as the degree of dentin demineralization, moisture control, and the application technique of the adhesive.

In minimally invasive dentistry, adhesive techniques are employed to enhance the preservation of natural tooth structure while achieving effective restorations. For instance, in cases of carious lesions, adhesive materials allow for the removal of only the affected dentin while preserving healthy tooth structure. This conservative approach is facilitated by the use of adhesives that bond directly to both the prepared tooth surface and the restorative material, ensuring a seamless integration and long-term durability of the restoration.

The application of adhesive dentistry extends beyond traditional restorations to include aesthetic enhancements, such as the placement of veneers and aesthetic bonding. These procedures rely heavily on the principles of adhesive bonding to achieve natural-looking results and maintain the integrity of the tooth structure. The precision of adhesive techniques is essential in ensuring that aesthetic restorations not only meet functional requirements but also blend harmoniously with the surrounding natural teeth.

In summary, adhesive dentistry has transformed modern restorative practices by providing techniques that emphasize tooth preservation and enhance the effectiveness of treatments. Understanding the types of dental adhesives, their applications, and the principles of bonding to enamel and dentin is essential for achieving successful outcomes in minimally invasive dentistry. As advancements in adhesive materials and techniques continue to evolve, practitioners are equipped with increasingly sophisticated tools to provide high-quality care while prioritizing the preservation of natural tooth structure.

Adhesive dentistry represents a cornerstone of modern restorative practices, bridging the gap between preserving natural tooth structure and achieving robust, functional restorations. The effectiveness of these restorative techniques hinges on the careful application of various bonding methods and the selection of appropriate dental adhesives, tailored to the specific requirements of each case. Understanding the nuances of these techniques is essential for any dental professional committed to the principles of minimally invasive dentistry.

The process of bonding begins with the preparation of the tooth surface, which is critical for achieving a strong and lasting connection between the restorative material and the natural tooth. This preparation varies based on whether the target surface is enamel or dentin, as each tissue type requires distinct handling to maximize adhesion.

Enamel, with its highly mineralized structure, presents a relatively straightforward bonding surface. The primary method for preparing enamel involves the use of acidic etchants. These acids, typically phosphoric acid, remove the outer layer of the enamel, exposing a rougher surface that enhances the mechanical retention of adhesives. The etching process creates microporosities that allow the adhesive to penetrate and form a solid bond. After etching, the application of a bonding resin further ensures that the adhesive material can adequately infiltrate these microporosities and establish a secure attachment. This well-established technique provides a high level of adhesion, particularly important for the success of composite restorations and other aesthetic enhancements.

Dentin, by contrast, is more complex due to its porous structure and the presence of dentinal tubules, which are channels filled with fluid and collagen fibers. The preparation of dentin involves a more nuanced approach to avoid compromising the tooth's structural integrity and its biological health. To bond effectively to dentin, the tooth surface must be conditioned to create a hybrid layer, a crucial element of the bonding process. This hybrid layer is formed by applying an adhesive that infiltrates the demineralized dentin and bonds with the underlying collagen network.

The bonding process to dentin is influenced by the type

of adhesive used and the specifics of the dentin surface preparation. Traditional etch-and-rinse systems involve a multi-step approach where an acidic etchant is first applied to the dentin to remove the mineral content and expose the collagen network. Following this, a primer is used to enhance the infiltration of adhesive resins into the demineralized dentin. Finally, a bonding resin is applied to seal the hybrid layer and provide a strong bond with the restorative material. This method is effective but requires careful technique to avoid issues such as over-etching, which can weaken the dentin or result in postoperative sensitivity.

Self-etch adhesives, which combine etching and priming in a single step, offer an alternative approach that simplifies the bonding process and reduces potential sources of error. These adhesives contain acidic components that simultaneously demineralize the dentin and promote bonding. Self-etch systems are particularly advantageous in clinical situations where a more conservative approach is beneficial, such as in cases involving minimal enamel loss or when working in challenging environments where moisture control is difficult. However, the effectiveness of self-etch adhesives can be influenced by the extent of dentin demineralization, which may affect their overall bonding performance.

Universal adhesives represent a significant advancement in adhesive dentistry, offering flexibility in their application and compatibility with various substrates. These adhesives can be used in both etch-and-rinse and self-etch modes, allowing practitioners to adapt their technique based on clinical needs. Universal adhesives are formulated to bond effectively to a range of materials, including both enamel and dentin, as well as restorative materials such as composites and ceramics. This versatility makes universal adhesives a valuable asset in modern dental practice, enabling practitioners to streamline their workflow and achieve reliable results across diverse clinical scenarios.

The successful application of adhesive dentistry is not limited to restorative procedures alone but extends to aesthetic treatments such as veneers and aesthetic bonding. In these applications, the precision and reliability of adhesive techniques are crucial for achieving natural-looking results and maintaining the integrity of the tooth structure. Veneers, for example, rely on the principles of adhesive bonding to ensure a secure and aesthetically pleasing attachment to the tooth surface. The use of high-quality adhesives and meticulous application techniques is essential for the long-term success of these treatments.

The principles of adhesive dentistry underscore the importance of a careful and informed approach to tooth preparation, adhesive application, and bonding. By understanding the different types of adhesives and their specific applications, dental professionals can enhance the effectiveness of minimally invasive treatments and provide high-quality care that aligns with the principles of tooth preservation and patient comfort. As advancements in adhesive materials and techniques continue to evolve, the field of adhesive dentistry will undoubtedly see further innovations that improve the outcomes of restorative and aesthetic procedures.

The effectiveness of adhesive dentistry is fundamentally tied to the quality and application of dental adhesives, which are designed to bond restorative materials to tooth structures with minimal invasion. This segment delves into the nuances of adhesive technology and its pivotal role in achieving durable and reliable restorations, focusing on the practical aspects and challenges encountered in clinical settings.

Among the various types of dental adhesives, the classification typically includes etch-and-rinse, self-etch, and universal adhesives. Each category has unique properties that influence its application and performance in bonding procedures. Etch-and-rinse adhesives, often regarded as the gold standard, involve a three-step process. This method starts with the application of a phosphoric acid etchant to remove the smear layer and demineralize the enamel or dentin, creating a roughened surface conducive to bonding. Following this, a primer is applied to infiltrate the demineralized areas and improve the wetting of the adhesive. Finally, a bonding resin is applied and light-cured to form a durable interface between the tooth structure and the restorative material. This well-established process is known for its high bond strength and reliability, though it demands precise execution and careful management of each step to avoid complications such as over-etching or inadequate bonding.

Self-etch adhesives offer a more streamlined approach by combining etching and priming in a single step. These adhesives contain acidic components that both demineralize the tooth surface and prepare it for bonding, simplifying the application process and reducing the number of steps involved. The advantage of self-etch adhesives lies in their ability to preserve more of the tooth's natural mineral content and reduce post-operative sensitivity. However, their effectiveness can vary depending on the type of dentin and the amount of demineralization required, making them a versatile yet sometimes less predictable option compared to traditional etch-and-rinse systems.

Universal adhesives represent a significant advancement in adhesive dentistry, designed to be adaptable to different bonding protocols. These adhesives can function in both etch-and-rinse and self-etch modes, offering flexibility based on clinical needs. They are formulated to bond to a variety of substrates, including enamel, dentin, and restorative materials such as composites and ceramics. The versatility of universal adhesives facilitates a more efficient workflow in clinical practice, as practitioners can use a single adhesive for multiple purposes. This adaptability, however, necessitates an understanding of the specific adhesive's characteristics and the appropriate technique for each application to ensure optimal results.

In addition to adhesive types, the principles of bonding to different tooth substrates—enamel and dentin—are crucial for successful restorative outcomes. Enamel bonding relies on the creation of a micro-mechanical interlocking between the adhesive and the etched enamel surface. The etching process enhances the surface area for bonding and improves the mechanical retention of the adhesive. Dentin bonding, conversely, involves a more complex interaction due to the presence of dentinal tubules and the need to establish a hybrid layer. The hybrid layer, formed by infiltrating the demineralized dentin with adhesive resin, serves as a crucial interface between the tooth and the restorative material. Effective bonding to dentin requires careful attention to the preparation and application techniques to avoid issues such as inadequate hybrid layer formation or contamination.

The longevity and effectiveness of adhesive restorations are influenced by several factors, including the proper selection of adhesives, meticulous application techniques, and appropriate post-operative care. Dental professionals must stay informed about advances in adhesive materials and techniques to maintain high standards of care and adapt to evolving clinical practices. Ongoing research and development in adhesive dentistry continue to enhance the performance and versatility of adhesive systems, offering new opportunities for improving the outcomes of restorative procedures.

Understanding the underlying principles of adhesive dentistry and mastering the application of various bonding techniques are fundamental for achieving successful, minimally invasive restorations. The ability to select and apply the appropriate adhesive system, based on the specific needs of each case, plays a crucial role in ensuring durable and aesthetically pleasing results. As the field of adhesive dentistry advances, continued education and hands-on experience will be essential for dental professionals to leverage the latest innovations and techniques in their practice.

CHAPTER 5: CARIES MANAGEMENT AND MINIMALLY INVASIVE RESTORATIONS

The management of dental caries is a critical component of modern dentistry, and the advent of minimally invasive techniques represents a paradigm shift from traditional methods. This chapter explores the contemporary approaches to caries management, emphasizing strategies that prioritize the preservation of natural tooth structure while effectively addressing decay. We will delve into methods for detecting caries, assessing risk, and employing conservative restorative materials.

Early and accurate detection of dental caries is pivotal in minimizing the extent of intervention required. Traditional diagnostic methods, such as visual examination and tactile assessment with dental explorers, remain essential. However, these techniques often fail to detect early carious lesions, which are crucial to identify for minimally invasive treatment. Advances in diagnostic technologies have significantly enhanced our ability to identify carious lesions at their inception. Digital radiography, with its high-resolution imaging capabilities, allows for the detection of caries that may not be visible to the naked eye. This technique reduces radiation exposure compared to traditional X-rays and provides detailed images that aid in assessing the extent of decay.

Additionally, fiber-optic transillumination and near-infrared light scanning are emerging technologies that offer non-invasive methods for detecting carious lesions. Fiber-optic transillumination works by passing a light through the tooth structure, with carious areas appearing as dark spots due to their decreased mineral content. Near-infrared light scanning, on the other hand, uses light absorption properties to detect carious dentin and assess its depth. Both methods contribute to a more comprehensive understanding of carious lesions, facilitating early intervention.

The principles of caries risk assessment play a crucial role in caries management. Risk assessment involves evaluating various factors that contribute to an individual's susceptibility to caries. These factors include dietary habits, oral hygiene practices, fluoride exposure, and socio-economic status. By understanding these risk factors, dental professionals can implement targeted preventive measures and tailor treatment plans to the individual's needs. For instance, patients with a high caries risk may benefit from increased fluoride treatments, more frequent professional cleanings, and dietary counseling to mitigate their risk.

Incorporating caries management by risk assessment into clinical practice aligns with the principles of minimally invasive dentistry, focusing on prevention and early intervention rather than extensive restoration. Caries management strategies may include the use of fluoride varnishes and sealants, which can help remineralize early carious lesions and prevent further progression. Fluoride varnishes, for example, release fluoride ions that enhance the tooth's ability to remineralize and resist decay. Sealants, often applied to the occlusal surfaces of molars, provide a physical barrier that protects against carious lesions by preventing food and bacteria from accumulating in the deep grooves of the teeth.

When carious lesions do require restoration, the focus shifts to utilizing conservative restorative materials that align with the principles of minimally invasive dentistry. These materials are designed to preserve as much natural tooth structure as possible while effectively addressing the decay. Composite resins are a popular choice due to their ability to bond to tooth structure and their aesthetic appearance, which blends seamlessly with the natural tooth color. Resin ionomer cements, which release fluoride, offer another conservative option, particularly for areas where aesthetic concerns are less critical.

The concept of minimally invasive restorations emphasizes the importance of precision and preservation. The goal is to remove only the decayed tissue while conserving healthy tooth structure, thereby maintaining the tooth's integrity and function. Techniques such as air abrasion and laser treatment are examples of minimally invasive methods that can be employed to prepare the tooth for restoration with minimal removal of healthy enamel and dentin. Air abrasion uses a stream of fine particles to remove carious tissue, while laser treatments offer precise removal of decayed tissue with minimal thermal damage to surrounding structures.

Post-restoration care is also an essential aspect of effective caries management. After placing a minimally invasive restoration, it is important to monitor the tooth for any signs of recurrent decay or complications. Regular follow-up appointments and ongoing patient education on maintaining oral hygiene are crucial for ensuring the longevity of the restoration and the overall health of the tooth.

In summary, the management of caries through minimally

invasive techniques represents a significant advancement in dental practice. By leveraging early detection technologies, assessing individual risk factors, and utilizing conservative restorative materials, dental professionals can effectively manage carious lesions while preserving the natural tooth structure. The integration of these principles into clinical practice not only enhances the efficacy of caries management but also aligns with the broader goals of minimally invasive dentistry, ultimately leading to improved patient outcomes and satisfaction.

In the realm of caries management and minimally invasive restorations, the focus extends beyond the immediate treatment of decay to encompass a broader preventive strategy. Effective management strategies integrate early detection, risk assessment, and conservative treatment approaches, all while emphasizing the preservation of natural tooth structure. This holistic approach is integral to minimizing the impact of dental caries on oral health.

The concept of early detection is central to minimally invasive dentistry. Traditional diagnostic methods, while foundational, often fall short in identifying carious lesions before they become clinically significant. Digital radiography has revolutionized caries detection by providing high-resolution images with reduced radiation exposure. This advanced imaging technique allows clinicians to observe carious lesions in detail, enabling accurate assessment and timely intervention. However, the utility of digital radiography is enhanced when combined with other diagnostic modalities.

Fiber-optic transillumination, for example, offers a non-invasive method to visualize carious lesions. This technique relies on light transmission through the tooth structure, revealing areas of demineralization that are otherwise invisible. Similarly, near-infrared light scanning provides insights into the depth and extent of carious lesions, offering a complementary tool to radiographic imaging. By utilizing a combination of diagnostic technologies, clinicians can achieve a comprehensive understanding of carious lesions, leading to more informed treatment decisions.

Beyond detection, assessing an individual's caries risk is crucial for effective management. Risk assessment involves evaluating various factors that contribute to an individual's susceptibility to caries. These factors include dietary habits, oral hygiene practices, fluoride exposure, and socio-economic status. By identifying patients at high risk, dental professionals can implement targeted preventive strategies tailored to their specific needs. For instance, patients with a high risk of caries may benefit from increased fluoride treatments and more frequent professional cleanings. Similarly, dietary counseling can help mitigate the effects of high-sugar diets that contribute to carious lesions.

The use of fluoride varnishes and dental sealants represents a proactive approach to caries prevention. Fluoride varnishes, applied topically, release fluoride ions that aid in the remineralization of early carious lesions. This remineralization process enhances the tooth's resistance to further decay and can effectively halt the progression of carious lesions. Dental sealants, typically applied to the occlusal surfaces of molars, provide a protective barrier that prevents food particles and bacteria from accumulating in the deep grooves of the teeth. Sealants are particularly beneficial for children and adolescents, who are more susceptible to caries in these areas.

When it comes to restorative treatment, minimally invasive techniques prioritize the preservation of natural tooth structure. Traditional restorative methods often involve extensive removal of healthy tooth tissue to access and treat carious lesions. In contrast, minimally invasive restorations focus on removing only the decayed tissue while conserving as much healthy enamel and dentin as possible. This approach not only maintains the tooth's structural integrity but also reduces the likelihood of future complications.

Composite resins are a prominent example of conservative restorative materials used in minimally invasive dentistry. These materials bond to tooth structure and can be color-matched to the natural tooth, offering both aesthetic and functional benefits. The application of composite resins involves a precise technique that includes the etching of enamel, the application of a bonding agent, and the placement of the resin material. This process ensures a strong bond between the restoration and the natural tooth, while preserving the tooth's original anatomy.

Resin ionomer cements, another conservative option, release fluoride ions over time, contributing to the long-term health of the tooth. These materials are particularly useful for areas where aesthetic concerns are less critical, such as in posterior teeth. Resin ionomers are applied in a similar manner to composite resins but offer the added benefit of fluoride release, which helps in the prevention of recurrent caries.

Minimally invasive techniques also encompass advanced methods such as air abrasion and laser treatment. Air abrasion uses a stream of fine particles to remove decayed tissue, minimizing the need for traditional drilling and reducing the removal of healthy tooth structure. Laser treatment, on the other hand, provides a precise means of removing decayed tissue with minimal thermal damage to surrounding structures. Both methods align with the principles of minimally invasive dentistry by focusing on precision and preservation.

Post-restoration care is essential for ensuring the longevity and effectiveness of minimally invasive treatments. After placing a restoration, it is important to monitor the tooth for signs of recurrent decay or other complications. Regular follow-up appointments, along with patient education on maintaining optimal oral hygiene practices, are critical for sustaining the health of the restored tooth and preventing future issues.

In conclusion, the management of dental caries through minimally invasive techniques represents a significant advancement in dental care. By integrating early detection technologies, risk assessment strategies, and conservative restorative materials, dental professionals can effectively manage carious lesions while preserving natural tooth structure. This comprehensive approach not only enhances the efficacy of caries management but also aligns with the broader goals of minimally invasive dentistry, ultimately contributing to improved patient outcomes and long-term oral health.

An integral aspect of managing dental caries through minimally invasive techniques involves not only the choice of restorative materials but also the approach to their application. Each treatment strategy and material used must be carefully selected based on the specific characteristics of the carious lesion and the overall condition of the tooth.

Adhesion technology plays a pivotal role in minimally invasive restorations. The success of a restoration largely depends on the ability of the chosen material to bond effectively to the tooth structure. Modern adhesive systems, which include etch-and-rinse, self-etch, and selective-etch techniques, are designed to enhance the bonding process. Etch-and-rinse systems involve applying an acidic etchant to the tooth surface, followed by rinsing and the application of a bonding agent. This technique provides a strong bond to both enamel and dentin but requires careful management to avoid over-etching, which can compromise the bonding strength.

Self-etch adhesives, in contrast, combine the etching and bonding steps into a single application. This approach simplifies the procedure and reduces the risk of over-etching while still providing a reliable bond. Self-etch systems are particularly useful in situations where minimal tooth preparation is needed, as they can be applied directly to the unprepared tooth surface. Selective-etch adhesives offer a middle ground, applying the etchant selectively to enamel while using a self-etch approach for dentin. This method takes advantage of the strong bonding properties to enamel while simplifying the process for dentin adhesion.

The choice of adhesive technique directly influences the longevity and effectiveness of the restoration. Ensuring a clean, dry surface and proper application technique are crucial for achieving optimal bonding. The use of bonding agents with antimicrobial properties can further enhance the durability of the restoration by reducing the risk of secondary caries and microbial invasion.

In addition to adhesive technologies, the choice of restorative materials is critical for maintaining the integrity of minimally invasive treatments. The primary goal is to use materials that replicate the natural properties of tooth structure while offering durability and resistance to decay. Composite resins, with their excellent aesthetic qualities and adaptability, are frequently used for fillings in both anterior and posterior teeth. Their ability to be color-matched to the natural tooth makes them a preferred choice for visible restorations.

For posterior restorations, where greater strength and wear resistance are required, materials such as resin-ionomer cements and glass ionomer cements are often utilized. These materials provide a durable bond and release fluoride, which contributes to the ongoing protection against caries. The choice between these materials often depends on the location of the restoration and the specific needs of the patient, such as their caries risk level and functional demands.

Minimally invasive techniques also extend to the management of carious lesions through non-invasive treatments. The use of therapeutic agents such as fluoride varnishes and calcium phosphates can help in the remineralization of early carious lesions. These treatments work by replenishing lost minerals and strengthening the tooth structure, potentially halting the progression of decay before it requires more invasive intervention.

Another promising approach in minimally invasive dentistry is the application of silver diamine fluoride (SDF). This compound has shown significant efficacy in arresting carious lesions by providing an antimicrobial effect and promoting remineralization. SDF is particularly useful in managing carious lesions in patients who are unable to undergo conventional restorative procedures due to medical conditions or high caries risk. Its application involves painting the solution onto the affected area, which then reacts with the tooth structure to halt decay and provide a protective layer.

As minimally invasive dentistry continues to evolve, ongoing research and development are focused on enhancing existing techniques and exploring new technologies. Advances in diagnostic tools, such as hyperspectral imaging and optical coherence tomography, promise to further refine caries detection and treatment planning. These technologies offer greater precision in identifying early-stage carious lesions and assessing the effectiveness of restorative treatments.

Additionally, the integration of artificial intelligence and machine learning into diagnostic and treatment planning processes is expected to revolutionize the field. These technologies can analyze large volumes of data to predict caries risk, optimize treatment protocols, and provide personalized patient care. The implementation of AI-driven tools in clinical practice will likely enhance decision-making processes, improve treatment outcomes, and support the continued advancement of minimally invasive techniques.

In summary, the management of dental caries through minimally invasive techniques represents a dynamic and evolving field within dentistry. By focusing on early detection, risk assessment, and the application of conservative restorative materials, dental professionals can effectively address carious lesions while preserving natural tooth structure. The integration of advanced diagnostic tools, adhesive technologies, and innovative restorative materials contributes to the overall success of minimally invasive treatments. As the field progresses, ongoing research and technological advancements will continue to shape the future of caries management and minimally invasive dentistry, ultimately improving patient care and outcomes.

CHAPTER 6: PREVENTIVE STRATEGIES AND PATIENT EDUCATION

Preventive strategies are foundational to the philosophy of minimally invasive dentistry, emphasizing the importance of maintaining oral health and avoiding the progression of dental diseases. This approach prioritizes proactive measures over reactive treatments, aiming to minimize the need for invasive procedures by focusing on prevention and early intervention.

One of the core elements of preventive dentistry is patient education. Educating patients about their oral health and the factors that contribute to dental issues is crucial for empowering them to take control of their oral hygiene. Effective patient education covers a range of topics, including proper brushing and flossing techniques, the impact of diet on dental health, and the importance of regular dental check-ups. By providing patients with the knowledge and tools they need, dental professionals can foster a collaborative approach to oral health that extends beyond the dental office.

Brushing and flossing are fundamental practices that play a critical role in preventing dental caries and periodontal disease. Dental professionals should emphasize the importance of brushing twice daily with fluoride toothpaste and flossing daily to remove plaque and food particles from between the teeth. Instruction on proper brushing techniques, such as using a soft-bristled brush and employing a gentle, circular motion, can help patients achieve a more thorough clean. Similarly, demonstrating effective flossing techniques ensures that patients can adequately clean the spaces between their teeth, where plaque accumulation is most likely to occur.

Dietary counseling is another vital component of preventive strategies. The consumption of sugary and acidic foods and beverages is a major risk factor for caries development. Dental professionals should advise patients on making dietary choices that promote oral health, such as consuming a balanced diet rich in fruits, vegetables, and whole grains while limiting sugary snacks and drinks. Educating patients about the impact of dietary habits on their oral health can help them make informed decisions that contribute to long-term dental well-being.

Regular dental check-ups and cleanings are essential for early detection and management of potential issues before they escalate into more significant problems. During these visits, dental professionals can perform comprehensive examinations, including the use of diagnostic technologies to identify early signs of carious lesions or periodontal disease. Professional cleanings help remove calculus and plaque that cannot be effectively addressed by routine home care, further reducing the risk of dental problems.

Fluoride treatments are a widely recognized preventive measure in dentistry. Fluoride is a mineral that helps strengthen tooth enamel and make it more resistant to acid attacks from plaque and dietary acids. Topical fluoride treatments, which are applied directly to the teeth in the form of gels, varnishes, or foams, provide an additional layer of protection against caries. Dental professionals often recommend fluoride treatments for patients at higher risk of caries, including children, individuals with a history of frequent caries, and those with reduced saliva flow.

Dental sealants are another effective preventive measure that protects the occlusal surfaces of the posterior teeth from caries. Sealants are thin, protective coatings applied to the grooves and pits of the molars and premolars, where carious lesions are most likely to develop. By sealing these areas, dental sealants prevent food particles and bacteria from accumulating in the deep fissures of the teeth. Sealants are particularly beneficial for children and adolescents, who are at a higher risk for caries due to their diet and oral hygiene habits. However, adults can also benefit from sealants, especially if they have deep fissures or are at increased risk for caries.

In addition to individual preventive measures, community-based programs play a significant role in promoting oral health on a broader scale. Public health initiatives, such as water fluoridation and school-based dental sealant programs, contribute to reducing the incidence of dental caries and improving overall oral health within communities. Dental professionals can support these initiatives by advocating for policies that promote access to preventive care and participating in community outreach programs that provide education and services to underserved populations.

Patient education and preventive strategies must be tailored to meet the specific needs of each individual. Personalized care plans that consider factors such as age, oral health history, and risk factors can help ensure that preventive measures are both effective and relevant. By engaging patients in their own oral health care and providing them with the knowledge and resources to make informed decisions, dental professionals can help create a proactive approach to maintaining dental health that aligns with the principles of minimally invasive dentistry.

In conclusion, preventive strategies and patient education are integral to the practice of minimally invasive dentistry. By focusing on education, preventive measures, and early intervention, dental professionals can help patients maintain optimal oral health and reduce the need for invasive treatments. The implementation of fluoride treatments, sealants, and dietary counseling, combined with regular dental check-ups, creates a comprehensive approach to preventing dental issues and promoting long-term dental well-being. Through collaborative efforts and personalized care, the goals of minimally invasive dentistry can be achieved, ultimately leading to improved oral health outcomes and a more positive dental experience for patients.

Preventive strategies are central to minimizing invasive dental procedures and preserving oral health through proactive care. This approach not only emphasizes the early detection of dental issues but also highlights the importance of maintaining optimal oral hygiene to prevent the onset of carious lesions and other dental conditions.

A critical aspect of preventive dentistry is the application of fluoride treatments. Fluoride, a naturally occurring mineral, fortifies tooth enamel, making it more resistant to demineralization caused by acidic environments. This resistance helps prevent the formation of cavities and supports the remineralization of early demineralized enamel. The effectiveness of fluoride in caries prevention is well-documented, with its application extending from professional treatments in the dental office to fluoride toothpaste and mouth rinses used at home. Regular fluoride applications can be particularly beneficial for individuals with a higher risk of caries, such as those with reduced saliva flow or a history of frequent dental issues.

Sealants represent another vital preventive measure in the fight against dental caries. These thin, protective coatings are applied to the occlusal surfaces of molars and premolars, where deep grooves and fissures are susceptible to plaque accumulation and carious activity. Sealants form a barrier that shields these vulnerable areas from bacteria and food particles, significantly reducing the risk of decay. This preventive intervention is especially advantageous for children and adolescents, as their posterior teeth are often more prone to carious lesions due to the complexity of their occlusal anatomy. However, adults with deep fissures or those at increased risk of caries can also benefit from sealant applications.

In addition to fluoride treatments and sealants, dietary counseling plays a pivotal role in preventive strategies. The relationship between diet and oral health is profound, with sugary and acidic foods being major contributors to carious disease. Dental professionals should educate patients about the impact of their dietary choices on dental health, advocating for a balanced diet rich in nutrients that support oral health while advising moderation of high-sugar and acidic foods. This education includes informing patients about the effects of frequent snacking and sipping on sugary beverages, which can lead to prolonged acid exposure and increased caries risk.

Effective oral hygiene practices are essential components of preventive care. Beyond the basic recommendations of brushing twice daily with fluoride toothpaste and flossing daily, dental professionals should provide guidance on advanced oral hygiene techniques. This might include the use of interdental brushes for patients with larger interdental spaces or the use of antimicrobial mouth rinses for individuals with specific oral health concerns. Personalized recommendations can enhance the effectiveness of home care routines and address individual needs, such as those related to orthodontic appliances or restorative work.

Patient education extends beyond individual care techniques to encompass the importance of regular dental visits. Routine dental check-ups and professional cleanings are crucial for the early detection of dental issues and the maintenance of oral health. During these visits, dental professionals can perform comprehensive examinations, including the use of advanced diagnostic tools, to identify potential problems before they develop into more severe conditions. Regular cleanings help to remove plaque and calculus that can contribute to periodontal disease and carious activity, further supporting preventive efforts.

The integration of preventive strategies into daily practice also involves leveraging technology to enhance patient care. Digital radiography, for instance, provides detailed images of dental structures with reduced radiation exposure compared to traditional film-based systems. These high-resolution images aid in the early detection of carious lesions, enabling timely intervention and minimizing the need for more invasive treatments. Similarly, intraoral cameras offer real-time visualization of oral conditions, facilitating patient education by allowing patients to see and understand the state of their oral health firsthand.

Preventive care must also address systemic factors that influence oral health. For example, the management of conditions such as dry mouth (xerostomia) is crucial, as reduced saliva flow can increase the risk of caries and other dental issues. Dental professionals should assess and address such conditions, potentially recommending saliva substitutes or stimulants as part of a comprehensive preventive strategy.

Incorporating preventive strategies into dental practice requires a collaborative approach involving both dental professionals and patients. Effective communication is key to ensuring that patients understand the rationale behind preventive measures and their role in maintaining oral health. By fostering a supportive environment that encourages patient engagement and adherence to preventive recommendations, dental professionals can help achieve better oral health outcomes and reduce the prevalence of dental diseases.

In conclusion, preventive strategies in minimally invasive dentistry encompass a range of measures designed to maintain oral health and minimize the need for invasive treatments. By focusing on fluoride treatments, dental sealants, dietary counseling, and effective oral hygiene practices, dental professionals can help prevent the onset of carious lesions and other dental issues. Regular dental visits and the use of advanced technologies further enhance the effectiveness of preventive care. Through comprehensive patient education and a collaborative approach, the goals of minimally invasive dentistry can be achieved, ultimately leading to improved long-term oral health and a reduction in the need for more invasive dental interventions.

The integration of preventive strategies into daily dental practice represents a significant shift towards proactive care in minimally invasive dentistry. It is not merely about the application of specific treatments but involves a comprehensive approach that emphasizes the importance of patient education and ongoing engagement in maintaining oral health.

One of the critical components of effective preventive strategies is the individualized patient care plan. Each patient presents unique oral health challenges and needs, requiring tailored preventive interventions. Dental professionals must assess various factors, including the patient's age, oral hygiene habits, dietary preferences, and risk factors such as genetic predisposition to dental diseases. This personalized approach ensures that preventive measures are not only relevant but also effective in addressing the specific needs of each patient.

Patient education is fundamental in fostering a preventative mindset. It is essential to convey information in a clear and accessible manner, ensuring that patients understand both the rationale behind preventive measures and how to implement them effectively in their daily routines. Educational efforts should extend beyond the mere provision of information to include practical demonstrations of proper brushing and flossing techniques. For instance, showing patients how to use dental floss correctly and discussing the benefits of various toothbrush types can significantly enhance their daily oral care routines.

Incorporating visual aids and interactive tools can further enhance patient understanding and compliance. For example, using digital simulations to demonstrate the effects of poor oral hygiene or the benefits of fluoride treatments can make the information more tangible and relatable. Additionally, providing patients with written materials or digital resources that they can review at home can reinforce the concepts discussed during their visits.

The role of technology in preventive dentistry cannot be overstated. Advances in digital tools and applications offer new opportunities for patient engagement and education. For instance, dental apps that provide reminders for brushing, flossing, and dental appointments can help patients stay on track with their oral health routines. Similarly, online resources and educational videos can offer additional support and guidance, complementing in-office education efforts.

An important aspect of preventive care involves monitoring and managing risk factors. Regular dental examinations are crucial for detecting early signs of potential problems, such as incipient carious lesions or the beginning stages of periodontal disease. Through the use of advanced diagnostic technologies, such as digital radiography and intraoral cameras, dental professionals can identify these issues before they progress, allowing for timely and less invasive interventions. Risk assessments also enable dental professionals to implement targeted preventive measures based on the patient's specific risk profile, such as increasing fluoride applications or recommending more frequent professional cleanings.

Preventive strategies should also address the broader context of oral health, including its impact on overall health and well-being. For example, the connection between oral health and systemic conditions such as cardiovascular disease, diabetes, and respiratory illnesses highlights the importance of maintaining good oral hygiene and regular dental care. Educating patients about these connections can underscore the relevance of preventive care and motivate them to adhere to recommended practices.

Moreover, preventive care must be continuously adapted to reflect emerging research and advancements in dental science. Staying informed about the latest developments, such as new materials and techniques for fluoride treatments, advancements in sealant technology, and evolving guidelines for caries management, allows dental professionals to provide the most current and effective preventive care. Continuing education and professional development are vital for maintaining expertise and integrating new knowledge into clinical practice.

Collaboration with other healthcare providers can also enhance preventive efforts. For example, working with pediatricians to promote oral health from an early age or coordinating with nutritionists to address dietary influences on dental health can create a more comprehensive approach to prevention. Such interdisciplinary collaboration helps address the broader determinants of oral health and fosters a more holistic approach to patient care.

Ultimately, the success of preventive strategies relies on a collaborative effort between dental professionals and patients. Establishing a trusting relationship and engaging patients in their own care is crucial for achieving long-term success. By providing clear information, personalized care plans, and ongoing support, dental professionals can empower patients to take an active role in their oral health, leading to better outcomes and a reduction in the need for more invasive treatments.

In conclusion, the focus on preventive strategies in minimally invasive dentistry highlights the importance of a proactive approach to oral health. Through patient education, the implementation of preventive measures, and the use of advanced technologies, dental professionals can effectively manage and mitigate the risk of dental issues. By fostering a collaborative and informed approach to oral care, the goals of minimally invasive dentistry can be realized, leading to improved patient outcomes and a more sustainable approach to dental health.

CHAPTER 7: TECHNIQUES FOR MINIMALLY INVASIVE RESTORATIVE DENTISTRY

Minimally invasive restorative dentistry seeks to achieve optimal outcomes while preserving as much of the natural tooth structure as possible. This chapter delves into the techniques that enable such a conservative approach, focusing on microdentistry, air abrasion, and laser dentistry. These methods are instrumental in minimizing the extent of intervention and enhancing patient comfort, aligning with the core principles of minimally invasive dentistry.

Microdentistry represents a significant advancement in the field, emphasizing the precision of restorative procedures. This technique involves the use of specialized instruments and technology to perform highly localized treatments with minimal disruption to the surrounding healthy tooth structure. Microdentistry typically utilizes magnification tools such as dental loupes or operating microscopes, which allow for greater visibility and precision during procedures. By magnifying the area of interest, clinicians can identify and address minute areas of decay or damage with exceptional accuracy. This precision not only improves the efficacy of the treatment but also minimizes the impact on healthy tooth structure, adhering to the principles of conservatism.

Air abrasion is another technique that has gained prominence in minimally invasive restorative dentistry. This method involves the use of a stream of compressed air mixed with fine abrasive particles to remove decayed or damaged tooth material. Unlike traditional drilling methods, which can be more invasive and produce significant vibration and heat, air abrasion offers a more gentle approach. The precision of air abrasion allows for the selective removal of decayed tissue while preserving healthy tooth structure. Additionally, air abrasion is often less intimidating for patients, as it reduces the noise and discomfort commonly associated with traditional dental drills. This technique is particularly effective for small to medium-sized cavities and is commonly used in conjunction with other minimally invasive techniques to achieve optimal restorative outcomes.

Laser dentistry introduces another dimension to minimally invasive restorative practices. Lasers provide a highly controlled and precise method for tissue removal and treatment, utilizing focused light energy to achieve various therapeutic effects. In restorative procedures, lasers can be employed to remove decayed tooth material, prepare the tooth surface for bonding, or even perform soft tissue procedures such as gingival contouring. The advantages of laser dentistry include reduced discomfort, less postoperative sensitivity, and a lower risk of infection. The precision of lasers allows for targeted treatment, minimizing the impact on adjacent healthy tissue and enhancing the overall outcome of the restorative procedure.

The integration of these techniques into restorative practice requires a comprehensive understanding of their respective applications and limitations. Each method offers unique benefits that contribute to the overarching goal of minimally invasive dentistry: preserving natural tooth structure while achieving effective restoration. The choice of technique often depends on the specific clinical scenario, including the location and extent of the damage, the patient's comfort, and the desired outcome. In many cases, a combination of these techniques may be employed to address various aspects of the restoration in a conservative manner.

Furthermore, the successful application of these techniques hinges on the skill and experience of the dental professional. Mastery of microdentistry, air abrasion, and laser dentistry requires specialized training and practice. Continuing education and hands-on experience are essential for maintaining proficiency and ensuring that these techniques are applied effectively. As technology continues to evolve, staying abreast of the latest advancements and incorporating them into clinical practice can further enhance the benefits of minimally invasive restorative dentistry.

The use of these advanced techniques also underscores the importance of patient-centered care. Minimally invasive approaches are designed not only to improve clinical outcomes but also to enhance the overall patient experience. By minimizing discomfort, reducing the need for extensive tooth removal, and shortening recovery times, these techniques align with the broader goals of patient satisfaction and well-being. Effective communication with patients about the benefits and limitations of these methods is crucial in ensuring their understanding and acceptance of the proposed treatment plan.

In summary, the techniques discussed in this chapter—microdentistry, air abrasion, and laser dentistry—play a pivotal role in advancing minimally invasive restorative dentistry. By focusing on precision, conserving natural tooth structure, and improving patient comfort, these methods embody the principles of a modern, conservative approach to dental restoration. As technology and techniques continue to evolve, the integration of these advanced methods into restorative practice will remain essential in achieving the goals of minimally invasive dentistry. Through ongoing education, skill development, and patient-centered care, dental professionals can effectively implement these techniques to enhance outcomes and contribute to the broader objectives of preserving and protecting natural tooth structure.

The application of microdentistry, air abrasion, and laser dentistry reflects a significant shift towards more conservative and less invasive restorative procedures in dental practice. Each technique offers distinct advantages in preserving natural tooth structure and enhancing patient comfort. To fully appreciate their impact, it is essential to understand how these techniques work in practical settings and the considerations for their effective use.

Microdentistry leverages high-precision tools to perform restorative procedures with minimal impact on healthy tooth structure. The core principle of microdentistry is to magnify the operative field, allowing for intricate work on small areas of decay or damage without the need for extensive drilling. This precision is achieved through the use of magnification devices such as dental loupes and operating microscopes. The enhanced visibility enables clinicians to identify and address microscopic lesions or defects that might be overlooked with the naked eye. In practice, microdentistry is particularly useful for treating early carious lesions or performing cosmetic enhancements where maintaining the integrity of the surrounding tooth structure is paramount.

Air abrasion provides a non-traditional method for cavity preparation and is an excellent example of a technique that aligns with the principles of minimally invasive dentistry. By utilizing a stream of compressed air mixed with fine abrasive particles, air abrasion gently removes decayed tissue from the tooth surface. This method offers several benefits over conventional drilling techniques. First, it produces minimal vibration and heat, reducing patient discomfort and anxiety associated with traditional dental drills. Second, air abrasion allows for a more selective removal of affected tissue, preserving healthy tooth structure and minimizing the overall extent of intervention. The technique is particularly effective for small to medium-sized cavities and can be used in conjunction with other restorative materials and methods to achieve a comprehensive treatment outcome.

Laser dentistry represents a cutting-edge advancement that enhances the minimally invasive approach by employing focused light energy for various therapeutic applications. Lasers can be used for hard tissue procedures, such as cavity preparation and tooth whitening, as well as soft tissue procedures, including gingival contouring and frenectomy. The precision of lasers allows for targeted treatment with minimal impact on surrounding tissues. Additionally, lasers often reduce the need for local anesthesia due to their ability to selectively interact with specific types of tissue, further improving patient comfort. The use of lasers in restorative procedures also facilitates quicker healing and reduces the risk of post-operative complications, aligning with the goals of minimally invasive dentistry.

Integrating these techniques into restorative practice requires a careful evaluation of the clinical scenario and a thorough understanding of each method's capabilities and limitations. For instance, while microdentistry excels in precision, it may not always be suitable for larger or more complex restorations. Similarly, air abrasion is most effective for specific types of decay and may not be the best choice for all restorative needs. Laser dentistry, while highly versatile, requires specialized training and equipment, and its application may vary based on the type of laser used and the specific procedure performed.

The effective use of these techniques also involves considering patient-specific factors. For example, patient anxiety, the location and extent of the carious lesion, and the desired aesthetic outcome all play a role in determining the most appropriate technique. By tailoring the approach to the individual patient's needs and preferences, dental professionals can enhance the overall treatment experience and achieve optimal outcomes.

In addition to their clinical applications, these techniques also reflect broader trends in dental technology and patient care. The move towards less invasive procedures aligns with a growing emphasis on patient comfort, safety, and long-term oral health. As technology continues to advance, new developments in microdentistry, air abrasion, and laser dentistry are likely to further refine these techniques and expand their applications. Staying informed about the latest research and innovations in these areas is crucial for dental professionals who aim to provide the highest standard of care.

Overall, the techniques discussed—microdentistry, air abrasion, and laser dentistry—represent significant advancements in minimally invasive restorative dentistry. Each technique contributes to a more conservative approach to dental care, emphasizing the preservation of natural tooth structure and enhancing patient comfort. By understanding and effectively implementing these methods, dental professionals can offer treatments that align with the principles of minimally invasive dentistry and contribute to improved clinical and patient outcomes. As the field continues to evolve, the integration of these techniques into everyday practice will remain a key component of delivering high-quality, patient-centered care.

The integration of microdentistry, air abrasion, and laser

dentistry into minimally invasive restorative dentistry represents a paradigm shift towards more conservative and patient-centered approaches. Each technique offers unique advantages that align with the overarching goals of preserving natural tooth structure and enhancing patient comfort, and their effective application requires an understanding of their specific strengths and limitations.

Microdentistry, as a precision-focused approach, utilizes advanced magnification tools to perform restorative work with an unparalleled degree of accuracy. The use of dental loupes and operating microscopes allows clinicians to visualize and address issues at a microscopic level, which is crucial for managing early-stage carious lesions and performing detailed cosmetic procedures. This heightened visibility enables practitioners to more accurately delineate the boundaries of decay, ensuring that only the affected tissue is removed while preserving the healthy tooth structure. This technique is especially beneficial for small, localized restorations where minimal intervention is critical. Moreover, the use of microdentistry not only improves the precision of restorations but also enhances the overall aesthetic outcomes by allowing for more detailed and refined work.

Air abrasion, on the other hand, offers a non-invasive method for cavity preparation that contrasts sharply with traditional drilling techniques. By using a stream of compressed air mixed with fine abrasive particles, air abrasion effectively removes decayed enamel and dentin with minimal discomfort and no heat generation. This method significantly reduces the need for local anesthesia, making it an appealing option for patients with dental anxiety or those undergoing minor restorative procedures. Air abrasion is particularly advantageous for treating small to medium-sized cavities and can be used in conjunction with adhesive materials to provide a durable and aesthetically pleasing restoration. The technique's ability to target only the affected areas helps maintain the integrity of the surrounding tooth structure, aligning with the principles of minimally invasive dentistry.

Laser dentistry, with its ability to precisely cut and shape both hard and soft tissues, represents a significant technological advancement in restorative procedures. Lasers offer a range of benefits, including reduced bleeding, minimized discomfort, and faster healing times compared to conventional methods. For hard tissue procedures, lasers can effectively remove carious tissue and prepare the tooth for restoration without the vibrations and noise associated with traditional drills. Soft tissue lasers are invaluable for procedures such as gingival contouring and the removal of overgrown tissue, providing a more comfortable and precise alternative to scalpel-based methods. The versatility of lasers allows for a broad spectrum of applications in restorative dentistry, making them a valuable addition to a minimally invasive practice.

However, the successful application of these techniques depends on various factors, including the clinical scenario, the specific needs of the patient, and the available technology. While microdentistry excels in precision, it may not be suitable for larger or more complex restorations where other techniques might be more effective. Air abrasion, although effective for certain types of cavities, may not address all forms of decay, especially those requiring more extensive intervention. Laser dentistry, while highly versatile, requires specialized equipment and training, and its use may vary based on the type of laser and the specific procedure being performed.

Incorporating these techniques into clinical practice also necessitates ongoing education and adaptation to emerging advancements. As technology continues to evolve, new innovations in microdentistry, air abrasion, and laser dentistry are likely to further refine these methods and expand their applications. Staying abreast of the latest research and technological developments is essential for dental professionals committed to providing the highest standard of care. This involves not only familiarizing oneself with new tools and techniques but also understanding their clinical implications and integrating them into treatment planning and patient management strategies.

Moreover, the integration of these minimally invasive techniques must be accompanied by a thorough understanding of their implications for patient care. This includes considering patient-specific factors such as anxiety levels, the extent and location of the dental issues, and the overall treatment goals. By tailoring the approach to each patient's unique needs and preferences, clinicians can enhance the efficacy of the restorative procedures and ensure a more positive patient experience.

In summary, the techniques of microdentistry, air abrasion, and laser dentistry each contribute to the goals of minimally invasive restorative dentistry by enabling more conservative, precise, and patient-friendly treatments. Their effective application requires a nuanced understanding of their respective advantages and limitations, as well as a commitment to continuous learning and adaptation. As the field of restorative dentistry continues to advance, these techniques will remain central to achieving optimal outcomes and advancing the practice of minimally invasive dentistry.

CHAPTER 8: THE ROLE OF BIOMATERIALS IN MINIMALLY INVASIVE DENTISTRY

The application of advanced biomaterials plays a pivotal role in minimally invasive dentistry, enabling practitioners to achieve restorative outcomes that are both effective and conservative. This chapter delves into the various types of biomaterials used in modern dental practice, including composite resins, glass ionomers, and dental ceramics. Each material offers distinct properties and advantages that align with the principles of minimally invasive techniques, which prioritize the preservation of natural tooth structure while providing durable and aesthetic restorations.

Composite resins have become a cornerstone of minimally invasive dentistry due to their versatility and ability to blend seamlessly with natural tooth structure. These materials are composed of a resin matrix reinforced with filler particles, which contribute to their strength and durability. Composite resins can be used for a wide range of restorative procedures, from filling small cavities to performing intricate cosmetic enhancements. Their key advantage lies in their ability to bond directly to the tooth structure through adhesive systems, which allows for the preservation of more natural enamel and dentin compared to traditional amalgam fillings.

The application of composite resins involves several critical steps, including cavity preparation, etching, bonding, and placement of the resin. The preparation process typically involves cleaning and conditioning the tooth surface to ensure a strong bond between the resin and the tooth. Etching, usually accomplished with an acid solution, creates a roughened surface that enhances the adhesive's ability to penetrate and form a strong bond. The bonding agent is then applied, followed by the composite resin, which is carefully shaped and cured using a special light. The result is a restoration that not only mimics the appearance of natural teeth but also provides functional benefits such as strength and wear resistance.

Glass ionomers, another important class of biomaterials, offer unique properties that make them particularly suitable for certain minimally invasive applications. These materials are composed of a glass powder and an organic acid, which react to form a gel-like substance that sets into a hard, durable material. One of the primary advantages of glass ionomers is their ability to release fluoride over time, which contributes to the prevention of secondary caries and enhances the overall health of the surrounding tooth structure. This fluoride release is especially beneficial in patients at higher risk for caries, making glass ionomers a valuable option for preventive and restorative purposes.

Glass ionomers are often used in areas where aesthetic considerations are less critical, such as in the restoration of posterior teeth or as base materials under other restorations. Their ability to bond chemically to both enamel and dentin eliminates the need for additional bonding agents, simplifying the restoration process. Additionally, the thermal compatibility of glass ionomers with tooth structure reduces the risk of post-operative sensitivity, making them a suitable choice for patients who may experience discomfort with other restorative materials.

Dental ceramics represent another advanced biomaterial that has significantly contributed to the field of minimally invasive dentistry. Ceramics are known for their exceptional aesthetic qualities, strength, and biocompatibility. They are commonly used in applications such as crowns, veneers, and inlays or onlays, where both functional and cosmetic outcomes are paramount. The use of ceramics allows for the creation of restorations that closely resemble natural tooth structure in color, translucency, and texture.

The fabrication of dental ceramics typically involves the use of computer-aided design and manufacturing (CAD/CAM) technology, which enhances the precision and fit of the final restoration. CAD/CAM systems allow for the creation of highly accurate digital impressions and the design of custom restorations that can be milled or printed with great detail. This technological advancement reduces the need for multiple appointments and minimizes the adjustments required, leading to a more efficient and patient-friendly process.

Despite their many advantages, each biomaterial also presents specific challenges and limitations that must be considered in clinical practice. Composite resins, while highly versatile, may require periodic maintenance and repair due to wear or staining over time. Glass ionomers, although beneficial for their fluoride release, may have lower mechanical strength compared to other materials, limiting their use in high-stress areas. Dental ceramics, while excellent for aesthetic restorations, can be more brittle and require careful handling and preparation to avoid fractures.

Incorporating these biomaterials into minimally invasive

restorative procedures involves a nuanced understanding of their properties and appropriate applications. Practitioners must evaluate factors such as the location and extent of the restoration, the patient's oral health and preferences, and the specific characteristics of each material to determine the most suitable approach. Additionally, ongoing advancements in biomaterials continue to expand the options available to clinicians, allowing for even more refined and effective minimally invasive techniques.

In summary, the role of biomaterials in minimally invasive dentistry is central to achieving successful restorative outcomes while adhering to the principles of conservation and patient comfort. Composite resins, glass ionomers, and dental ceramics each offer distinct benefits that enhance the practice of minimally invasive dentistry. Understanding the properties, applications, and limitations of these materials enables practitioners to provide high-quality care that aligns with the goals of preserving natural tooth structure and promoting overall oral health.

The integration of advanced biomaterials into minimally invasive dentistry represents a significant evolution in restorative practices. These materials are specifically designed to support techniques that aim to preserve natural tooth structure while achieving effective and durable restorations. To fully appreciate their impact, it is essential to understand how these biomaterials work, their specific properties, and their clinical applications.

Composite resins, among the most widely used biomaterials, offer remarkable versatility and adaptability in restorative procedures. Composed of a resin matrix combined with inorganic filler particles, these materials are formulated to mimic the natural appearance and mechanical properties of dental tissues. The resin matrix provides flexibility and adhesion, while the fillers enhance the strength and durability of the material. This combination allows for a range of applications, from small fillings to extensive restorations, all while preserving the maximum amount of healthy tooth structure.

One of the primary advantages of composite resins is their ability to bond directly to tooth enamel and dentin. This adhesion is facilitated by a bonding agent that chemically interacts with the tooth surface and the resin. The bonding process begins with the application of an etching agent, which creates microscopic roughness on the enamel or dentin surface, increasing the surface area for adhesion. Following this, a primer and adhesive are applied, which penetrate the etched surface and form a strong bond with the composite resin. This technique not only enhances the retention of the restoration but also reduces the need for extensive tooth preparation, aligning with the principles of minimally invasive dentistry.

The adaptability of composite resins extends to their color-matching capabilities, making them particularly useful for aesthetic restorations. The ability to customize the shade and translucency of the resin ensures that restorations blend seamlessly with the natural dentition. Additionally, advancements in nanotechnology have led to the development of high-performance composites with improved wear resistance and reduced susceptibility to staining. These innovations contribute to the longevity and effectiveness of composite restorations, further supporting the goals of minimally invasive treatment.

Glass ionomers, another crucial category of biomaterials, offer unique properties that complement minimally invasive techniques. These materials are known for their chemical bond to tooth structure and their ability to release fluoride over time. The fluoride release is particularly beneficial in preventing secondary caries, making glass ionomers a valuable option for high-risk patients or areas where additional caries protection is desired. The chemical bond formed with the tooth structure eliminates the need for additional bonding agents, streamlining the restoration process.

Glass ionomers are also characterized by their ease of use and compatibility with various restorative scenarios. They can be used as base materials under other restorations or for filling small cavities in areas where aesthetic considerations are less critical. Their thermal compatibility with tooth structure helps minimize post-operative sensitivity, providing additional comfort for patients. However, their mechanical properties, while adequate for many applications, may not be as strong as those of other materials, which can limit their use in high-stress areas.

Dental ceramics are another advanced biomaterial that has revolutionized restorative dentistry, particularly in applications where both strength and aesthetics are paramount. Ceramics are known for their excellent biocompatibility, durability, and ability to closely replicate the natural appearance of teeth. They are commonly used in crowns, veneers, and inlays or onlays, where their superior aesthetic qualities and mechanical strength are essential.

The development of computer-aided design and manufacturing (CAD/CAM) technology has significantly enhanced the precision and efficiency of ceramic restorations. CAD/CAM systems enable the creation of highly accurate digital impressions, which are used to design custom restorations that can be milled or printed with exceptional detail. This technology reduces the need for multiple visits and adjustments, streamlining the restorative process and improving patient satisfaction.

Despite their many advantages, dental ceramics present

certain challenges. Their brittleness requires careful handling during preparation and placement to avoid fractures. Additionally, the initial cost of ceramic restorations can be higher compared to other materials, which may influence their use in certain clinical scenarios. However, the long-term benefits of ceramics, including their durability and aesthetic appeal, often justify the investment.

In summary, the role of biomaterials in minimally invasive dentistry is integral to achieving successful restorative outcomes while adhering to the principles of conservation and patient comfort. Composite resins, glass ionomers, and dental ceramics each offer distinct benefits that enhance the practice of minimally invasive techniques. By understanding the properties, applications, and limitations of these materials, clinicians can make informed decisions that align with the goals of preserving natural tooth structure and promoting overall oral health. The continued advancement in biomaterials promises to further refine and expand the possibilities for minimally invasive restorative procedures, ultimately improving patient outcomes and satisfaction.

In addition to composite resins, glass ionomers, and dental ceramics, other advanced biomaterials play significant roles in minimally invasive dentistry. These include newer innovations such as resin ionomer cements, hybrid materials, and bioactive glass. Each of these materials has been developed to address specific clinical needs, offering further refinement to the principles of minimally invasive techniques.

Resin ionomer cements combine the properties of glass ionomers with those of composite resins. These materials are designed to enhance the strength and wear resistance of traditional glass ionomer cements while maintaining their ability to release fluoride. The resin component improves the bond to tooth structure and increases the overall mechanical performance. This makes resin ionomer cements particularly useful for restorative procedures in areas subjected to moderate to high mechanical stress, such as posterior teeth. Their fluoride-releasing capability continues to offer a preventive advantage, reducing the risk of secondary caries, while the enhanced physical properties provide a durable restoration.

Hybrid materials represent another advance in biomaterial technology, combining different types of resins or incorporating fillers to achieve a balance of desirable properties. For instance, hybrid composites often mix different types of fillers to improve both strength and polishability. These materials are engineered to meet the varying demands of clinical practice, including esthetics, wear resistance, and ease of manipulation. By tailoring the material properties to specific applications, hybrid materials contribute to more conservative restorative approaches, reducing the need for extensive tooth preparation and enhancing patient outcomes.

Bioactive glass is an innovative biomaterial with unique benefits for minimally invasive dentistry. It is composed of silicate-based materials that react with the biological environment to form a hydroxycarbonate apatite layer, which integrates with tooth structure and bone. This bioactivity allows bioactive glass to promote the remineralization of enamel and dentin, effectively combating early stages of carious lesions and enhancing the durability of restorations. Its ability to release calcium, phosphate, and fluoride ions further supports the repair of demineralized tooth structure and reduces the risk of secondary caries. Bioactive glass can be used in various applications, including as a component in restorative materials or as a direct application in areas at risk of carious development.

The selection of appropriate biomaterials for minimally invasive procedures depends on several factors, including the location and extent of the restoration, the patient's oral health, and the specific mechanical and esthetic requirements of the case. Clinicians must consider these factors carefully to choose the most suitable material for each situation. The decision-making process often involves evaluating material properties such as bond strength, wear resistance, esthetic matching, and fluoride release, as well as assessing the clinical context and patient preferences.

Future developments in biomaterial science are likely to further enhance the capabilities of minimally invasive dentistry. Research into new materials and technologies continues to advance, focusing on improving the performance, biocompatibility, and longevity of restorative materials. For instance, ongoing studies are exploring the use of nanotechnology to create materials with superior mechanical properties and enhanced interaction with biological tissues. Additionally, advancements in material processing techniques, such as 3D printing and digital fabrication, promise to offer more precise and efficient restorative solutions.

As minimally invasive dentistry evolves, the integration of advanced biomaterials will continue to play a critical role in achieving optimal outcomes. The emphasis on preserving natural tooth structure, minimizing intervention, and enhancing patient comfort aligns with the broader goals of modern dental practice. By leveraging the unique properties of various biomaterials, clinicians can provide effective and aesthetically pleasing restorations while adhering to the principles of minimal invasiveness.

In summary, the role of biomaterials in minimally invasive dentistry is pivotal in advancing restorative practices. Composite resins, glass ionomers, dental ceramics, resin ionomer cements, hybrid materials, and bioactive glass each contribute to the conservative approach that characterizes minimally invasive techniques. These materials offer a range of properties and applications that support the preservation of tooth structure and the achievement of durable, esthetic restorations. As the field of biomaterial science continues to progress, it will further refine and expand the possibilities for minimally invasive dentistry, ultimately benefiting both clinicians and patients.

CHAPTER 9: MANAGEMENT OF NON-CARIOUS TOOTH STRUCTURE LOSS

The management of non-carious tooth structure loss is an essential aspect of minimally invasive dentistry, addressing conditions such as erosion, abrasion, and attrition. Each of these issues presents unique challenges that require tailored diagnostic, preventive, and restorative approaches to effectively preserve tooth structure while maintaining oral health.

Erosion refers to the loss of tooth structure due to chemical processes, often as a result of acidic foods, beverages, or gastrointestinal conditions like acid reflux. The diagnostic approach for erosion involves a comprehensive assessment of dietary habits, medical history, and clinical examination. Dentists may use a combination of visual inspection, tactile examination, and advanced diagnostic tools such as digital imaging to evaluate the extent and severity of erosive damage. It is crucial to identify the underlying causes of erosion to implement appropriate preventive measures.

Preventive strategies for erosion focus on reducing the

impact of acid on tooth surfaces. This can include dietary modifications, such as reducing the intake of acidic foods and beverages, and recommending the use of fluoride treatments or remineralizing agents to strengthen enamel. Additionally, patients may be advised to rinse their mouth with water after consuming acidic substances and to avoid brushing immediately after acid exposure, as this can further damage softened enamel.

When restorative treatment is necessary for erosion, minimally invasive options are preferred to conserve as much natural tooth structure as possible. Techniques such as the application of dental veneers or bonding materials can be used to address cosmetic concerns and restore function. These materials should be selected based on their ability to withstand the erosive environment while providing a natural appearance and adequate protection for the underlying tooth structure.

Abrasion, another form of non-carious tooth structure loss, occurs due to mechanical wear from external sources, such as aggressive tooth brushing or abrasive toothpaste. The diagnosis of abrasion involves evaluating the wear patterns on teeth and assessing the patient's oral hygiene habits. In cases where abrasion is identified, it is essential to educate the patient on proper brushing techniques, including the use of a soft-bristled toothbrush and non-abrasive toothpaste.

Preventive measures for abrasion include modifying brushing habits and using protective devices, such as custom-made night guards, if bruxism is contributing to tooth wear. Additionally, adjusting the patient's oral hygiene routine and recommending the use of gentle, fluoride-containing products can help mitigate further abrasion.

Restorative treatments for abrasion aim to repair and protect worn areas while preserving as much tooth structure as possible. Composite resins or dental bonding materials can be applied to affected areas to restore tooth integrity and function. These materials should be selected based on their durability and compatibility with the patient's dental and aesthetic needs.

Attrition, the third type of non-carious tooth structure loss, results from the mechanical wear of teeth due to tooth-to-tooth contact, often associated with bruxism or malocclusion. Diagnosing attrition involves examining wear facets and assessing occlusal relationships. In addition to a clinical examination, dentists may use diagnostic tools such as occlusal analysis to evaluate the extent of wear and identify contributing factors.

Preventive strategies for attrition focus on managing the underlying causes of excessive tooth wear. This may include recommending occlusal splints to protect teeth from bruxism, adjusting the occlusion to correct malalignment, and providing patient education on stress management techniques if bruxism is stress-related. Early intervention can help prevent further damage and preserve tooth structure.

For cases of significant attrition that require restorative intervention, options such as dental crowns or onlays may be considered. Minimally invasive techniques, such as indirect restorations that require minimal tooth preparation, can be employed to restore function and esthetics while conserving as much healthy tooth structure as possible.

The overarching goal in managing non-carious tooth structure loss is to implement strategies that address both the symptoms and underlying causes while minimizing intervention. By adopting a comprehensive approach that includes accurate diagnosis, effective prevention, and conservative restorative techniques, dental practitioners can help patients maintain optimal oral health and preserve their natural tooth structure.

In summary, the management of non-carious tooth structure loss requires a multifaceted approach involving accurate diagnosis, preventive measures, and minimally invasive restorative options. Erosion, abrasion, and attrition each present distinct challenges that necessitate tailored strategies to preserve tooth structure and maintain oral health. By focusing on early intervention and conservative treatment, dental professionals can effectively manage these conditions and enhance patient outcomes.

When addressing non-carious tooth structure loss, it is crucial to understand how each condition affects the tooth and the available strategies to manage and treat these conditions effectively. As previously discussed, erosion, abrasion, and attrition each present unique challenges, but they also offer opportunities for innovative approaches to maintain tooth health and structure.

Erosion, characterized by the chemical degradation of tooth enamel due to acidic exposure, necessitates a nuanced approach to both prevention and treatment. The role of dietary counseling cannot be overstated in managing erosion. Patients should be guided to limit their consumption of acidic foods and beverages, which are known to significantly contribute to enamel erosion. For those with gastrointestinal conditions that exacerbate erosion, such as acid reflux, it is vital to address these underlying issues in tandem with dental treatments.

Professional interventions for erosion may include the application of fluoride varnishes or remineralizing agents that can help restore lost minerals and strengthen the enamel. In cases where erosion has progressed to the point where restorative work is needed, dentists might consider the use of dental bonding agents or composite resins. These materials are adept at providing a protective layer over the eroded surface while blending seamlessly with the natural tooth structure. The choice of restorative material is influenced by factors such as the extent of erosion, the location of the affected teeth, and patient preferences.

Abrasion, resulting from mechanical wear due to factors like improper brushing techniques, often requires modifications to the patient's oral hygiene routine. Education on proper brushing techniques is essential. Patients should be encouraged to use a soft-bristled toothbrush and to apply gentle brushing strokes. The use of toothpaste with a lower abrasive index can also minimize further enamel wear. In cases where abrasion has caused significant tooth loss, restorative options such as bonded restorations or veneers may be employed to restore the tooth's function and appearance while preserving as much of the natural tooth structure as possible.

Attrition, the wear and tear resulting from tooth-to-tooth contact, is frequently associated with bruxism. The management of attrition often involves a multidisciplinary approach. Addressing bruxism requires not only dental intervention but also potentially behavioral or medical management. The use of occlusal splints or night guards can protect the teeth from further wear. Additionally, patients may benefit from stress management techniques or orthodontic treatments if malocclusion is contributing to the attrition. When restorative work is necessary, options like crowns or overlays can be used to rehabilitate severely worn teeth. Minimally invasive techniques are preferred to ensure that the remaining healthy tooth structure is preserved.

For each of these conditions—erosion, abrasion, and attrition—early diagnosis and intervention are key to preventing further damage and maintaining oral health. Regular dental check-ups and vigilant patient self-care play pivotal roles in managing non-carious tooth structure loss. Advanced diagnostic tools, such as digital imaging and clinical examination, provide critical insights into the extent of the damage and help in formulating an effective treatment plan.

In addition to direct restorative treatments, preventive measures are fundamental in managing non-carious tooth structure loss. This involves not only addressing the immediate needs of the patient but also implementing long-term strategies to prevent recurrence. Patients should be educated about the importance of maintaining good oral hygiene practices, using fluoride-containing products, and seeking regular dental evaluations.

Furthermore, collaboration between dental professionals and patients is essential in devising personalized care plans. Understanding the patient's lifestyle, dietary habits, and any underlying medical conditions can help tailor preventive and restorative strategies to their specific needs. This comprehensive approach ensures that treatment is not only effective but also sustainable over the long term.

Ultimately, the management of non-carious tooth structure loss underscores the importance of a conservative and patient-centered approach. By emphasizing early intervention, preventive care, and minimally invasive restorative options, dental professionals can effectively address erosion, abrasion, and attrition while preserving as much natural tooth structure as possible. This approach not only enhances patient outcomes but also contributes to the overall goal of maintaining optimal oral health throughout the lifespan.

Effective management of non-carious tooth structure loss requires a thorough understanding of the interplay between diagnosis, prevention, and restoration. Each of these elements contributes to preserving tooth integrity and functionality while minimizing the impact of conditions such as erosion, abrasion, and attrition.

In diagnosing non-carious tooth structure loss, a comprehensive approach is crucial. Clinicians utilize a combination of visual examination, patient history, and advanced diagnostic tools to assess the extent of tooth damage. Digital radiography, for instance, offers high-resolution images that aid in detecting subtle changes in tooth structure and underlying issues not immediately visible. Additionally, intraoral cameras provide detailed images of the tooth's surface, facilitating a more precise evaluation of wear patterns and damage. These diagnostic tools not only enhance the accuracy of the diagnosis but also enable clinicians to monitor changes over time and adjust treatment plans accordingly.

Preventive strategies play a vital role in mitigating non-carious tooth structure loss. For erosion, preventive measures extend beyond dietary modifications to include the use of remineralizing agents and fluoride treatments. Fluoride helps in the re-mineralization of enamel and makes it more resistant to further acid attacks. Regular application of fluoride varnishes, particularly for patients with high caries risk, can significantly reduce the progression of erosion. In addition, recommending the use of neutral or alkaline mouth rinses can help neutralize acids and protect enamel.

In managing abrasion, patient education on proper brushing techniques is essential. Dentists should emphasize the importance of using a soft-bristled toothbrush and non-abrasive toothpaste. Moreover, advising patients to avoid excessive force while brushing and to replace their toothbrush regularly can help prevent further enamel wear. For patients with a history of abrasive wear, it is beneficial to incorporate regular check-ups to monitor any potential damage and provide timely interventions.

Attrition management often involves addressing the

underlying causes, such as bruxism, which can lead to significant tooth wear. The use of occlusal splints or night guards is a common preventive measure to protect teeth from grinding forces. Additionally, behavioral modifications, such as stress management or orthodontic adjustments, may be necessary to address the root causes of bruxism. For patients with severe attrition, restorative treatments such as crowns or overlays are considered to restore tooth function and protect the remaining tooth structure.

When restorative intervention is necessary, minimally invasive techniques are preferred to preserve as much of the natural tooth structure as possible. For erosion, composite resins and glass ionomer cements are often used to provide a protective layer over the eroded surface. These materials not only restore tooth structure but also blend aesthetically with natural teeth. In cases of abrasion, bonded restorations or veneers may be employed to restore the tooth's appearance and function while minimizing additional tooth preparation. For attrition, conservative restorative options, such as partial crowns or onlays, can rehabilitate worn teeth while maintaining the integrity of the remaining structure.

The integration of advanced biomaterials in restorative practices is crucial for achieving optimal results with minimal intervention. Materials such as high-strength composites, glass ionomers, and dental ceramics offer excellent durability and esthetics while being minimally invasive. These biomaterials are selected based on their compatibility with the tooth structure, their mechanical properties, and their ability to bond effectively to the tooth surface. The choice of material is tailored to the specific needs of the patient, considering factors such as the location and extent of tooth damage, as well as patient preferences.

Collaboration between dental professionals and patients is essential in developing an effective management plan for non-carious tooth structure loss. Open communication ensures that patients are informed about their condition, the available treatment options, and the importance of adhering to preventive measures. Regular follow-up appointments allow for monitoring of the condition and the effectiveness of the chosen interventions. This ongoing dialogue helps in making timely adjustments to the treatment plan and reinforces the patient's role in maintaining oral health.

In summary, the management of non-carious tooth structure loss involves a multifaceted approach that includes accurate diagnosis, preventive care, and minimally invasive restorative techniques. By leveraging advanced diagnostic tools, educating patients, and employing innovative biomaterials, dental professionals can effectively address erosion, abrasion, and attrition while preserving as much natural tooth structure as possible. This comprehensive approach not only enhances the longevity and function of the affected teeth but also supports overall oral health and patient well-being.

CHAPTER 10: MINIMALLY INVASIVE ENDODONTICS

Minimally invasive endodontics represents a significant shift from traditional root canal treatments, aiming to preserve as much natural tooth structure as possible while still effectively addressing the underlying issues within the tooth. This approach integrates advanced technologies, refined techniques, and innovative materials to enhance the efficacy and comfort of endodontic procedures.

The foundation of minimally invasive endodontics lies in the principle of conserving tooth structure. Traditional endodontic procedures often required extensive removal of tooth structure to access the root canals, which could compromise the structural integrity of the tooth. In contrast, minimally invasive techniques emphasize precision and conservation, aiming to achieve effective treatment with minimal intervention. This philosophy is guided by advancements in diagnostic and therapeutic technologies, which enable more accurate and less invasive access to the root canal system.

One of the key advancements in minimally invasive endodontics is the development of refined endodontic instruments. Modern endodontic handpieces and rotary instruments are designed to be more efficient and less aggressive, allowing for precise canal shaping with minimal removal of tooth structure. These instruments are typically smaller and more flexible, which helps in navigating the complex anatomy of root canals while preserving the surrounding dentin. The use of nickel-titanium (NiTi) rotary files, for example, has revolutionized endodontic practice by providing enhanced flexibility and durability, which is critical for minimally invasive procedures.

Another significant advancement is the application of advanced imaging techniques. Cone beam computed tomography (CBCT) provides three-dimensional imaging that allows for a detailed view of the root canal system, including its curvature, diameter, and any accessory canals. This comprehensive visualization aids in precise diagnosis and treatment planning, enabling clinicians to tailor their approach to the specific anatomy of each tooth. By understanding the intricacies of the canal system before commencing treatment, practitioners can avoid unnecessary removal of tooth structure and focus on areas requiring intervention.

The utilization of magnification and illumination in minimally invasive endodontics further enhances precision. Operating microscopes and loupes equipped with high-intensity lighting offer a magnified view of the tooth structure, improving the accuracy of canal cleaning and shaping. This enhanced visualization is particularly beneficial in identifying and treating narrow or calcified canals, which might otherwise be missed with conventional techniques. The combination of magnification and illumination ensures that only the necessary tooth structure is accessed and treated, reducing the risk of iatrogenic damage.

The introduction of modern irrigation techniques also supports the minimally invasive approach. Effective cleaning and disinfection of the root canal system are crucial for the success of endodontic therapy. Newer irrigation protocols and the use of ultrasonic or sonic activation devices enhance the penetration and efficacy of irrigants, ensuring that even complex canal systems are thoroughly debrided. This improved irrigation not only aids in the removal of debris but also reduces the need for aggressive mechanical instrumentation.

In terms of materials, minimally invasive endodontics benefits from advancements in biocompatible and adhesive materials. Modern root canal sealers and obturating materials are designed to provide superior sealing and adhesion while requiring less aggressive preparation of the canal space. Resilon, a thermoplastic root canal filling material, is an example of such innovation, offering excellent adaptability to the canal anatomy and enhancing the overall quality of the root canal seal. The use of these advanced materials minimizes the risk of post-treatment complications and contributes to the long-term success of the endodontic procedure.

Conservative approaches in endodontics are complemented by improved techniques in post-treatment restoration. Minimally invasive endodontics often involves the use of bonded composites or indirect restorations, which provide strength and protection to the treated tooth without necessitating extensive removal of remaining tooth structure. These restorative options are designed to support the integrity of the tooth while preserving as much of the natural dentin as possible, aligning with the overarching goal of minimally invasive dentistry.

Patient management and comfort are also integral to minimally invasive endodontics. Techniques such as careful anesthesia administration and the use of biocompatible materials contribute to a more comfortable experience for the patient. Minimizing discomfort and promoting a quicker recovery are key aspects of the conservative approach, enhancing patient satisfaction and compliance.

In conclusion, minimally invasive endodontics represents a paradigm shift in root canal therapy, focusing on preserving tooth structure and improving patient outcomes through advanced techniques and technologies. By integrating refined instruments, enhanced imaging, magnification, improved irrigation, and advanced materials, this approach ensures effective treatment with minimal intervention. The emphasis on conservation aligns with the broader principles of minimally invasive dentistry, ultimately contributing to the long-term health and function of the treated tooth.

Minimally invasive endodontics is characterized by its emphasis on reducing the extent of tooth preparation while still achieving effective and durable outcomes. This philosophy aligns with the broader goals of minimally invasive dentistry, focusing on preserving as much natural tooth structure as possible. The integration of advanced tools, techniques, and materials has played a pivotal role in advancing these conservative practices.

The refinement of endodontic instruments has been a cornerstone of minimally invasive techniques. Historically, endodontic treatments required extensive and often aggressive shaping of the root canal system, which could compromise the tooth's structural integrity. Modern rotary and reciprocating systems have transformed this aspect of endodontics. These newer instruments are designed with advanced metallurgy and precision engineering, allowing for more controlled and less invasive canal preparation. Nickel-titanium (NiTi) files, for instance, offer enhanced flexibility and resistance to fracture, which is crucial for navigating complex root canal anatomy with minimal tooth removal.

Furthermore, advancements in imaging technology have significantly influenced minimally invasive endodontics. Cone beam computed tomography (CBCT) provides a three-dimensional view of the tooth, offering detailed insights into the root canal system's structure. This enhanced visualization allows for precise planning and execution of endodontic procedures, minimizing the need for exploratory drilling and extensive tooth preparation. With CBCT, clinicians can identify variations in canal anatomy and tailor their approach accordingly, reducing the risk of over-preparation and preserving the tooth's natural structure.

In conjunction with improved instrumentation and imaging, the development of enhanced irrigation techniques has contributed to the minimally invasive paradigm. Effective irrigation is crucial for cleaning and disinfecting the root canal system, which is essential for the success of the treatment. Modern irrigation protocols, including the use of ultrasonic or sonic activation, ensure that irrigants reach all parts of the canal system, effectively removing debris and bacteria. This reduces the need for aggressive mechanical instrumentation and helps maintain the integrity of the surrounding dentin.

The role of biocompatible and adhesive materials in minimally invasive endodontics cannot be overstated. Contemporary endodontic sealers and filling materials are designed to provide excellent adhesion and sealing properties with minimal impact on the tooth structure. For example, bioceramic sealers and root canal sealants offer superior biocompatibility and durability while requiring less aggressive canal shaping. These materials contribute to a hermetic seal, preventing the ingress of bacteria and promoting the long-term success of the root canal treatment.

Minimally invasive endodontics also emphasizes conservative post-treatment restoration strategies. The choice of restorative materials and techniques is crucial for maintaining the tooth's structural integrity and functionality. Adhesive composites and indirect restorations, such as crowns and onlays, are often preferred for their ability to bond to the remaining tooth structure and provide strength without necessitating extensive removal of healthy dentin. These restorative options align with the minimally invasive philosophy by preserving as much of the natural tooth as possible while still achieving functional and esthetic results.

Patient comfort and management are integral to the success of minimally invasive endodontic procedures. Advances in local anesthesia techniques and materials contribute to a more comfortable experience for the patient. Precise administration of anesthesia and the use of biocompatible materials help minimize discomfort during and after the procedure, enhancing patient satisfaction and promoting a smoother recovery.

In addition to technological advancements, the principles of minimally invasive endodontics are supported by a growing body of clinical evidence and research. Studies have demonstrated that conservative approaches, when applied correctly, can yield outcomes comparable to or even superior to traditional techniques, with the added benefit of preserving natural tooth structure. This evidence reinforces the importance of adopting minimally invasive practices and encourages ongoing innovation and refinement in the field.

Overall, the principles of minimally invasive endodontics are grounded in a commitment to conserving tooth structure while delivering effective and reliable treatment. The integration of advanced instruments, imaging technology, improved irrigation techniques, and biocompatible materials underscores the evolution of endodontic practice toward more conservative and patient-centered approaches. By focusing on precision, conservation, and patient comfort, minimally invasive endodontics represents a significant advancement in the field, aligning with the broader goals of minimally invasive dentistry and contributing to the long-term health and function of the treated tooth.

The landscape of endodontics has been significantly transformed by the principles of minimally invasive dentistry, with a focus on preserving as much natural tooth structure as possible while achieving successful treatment outcomes. This approach emphasizes not only the advancement of techniques and materials but also a paradigm shift in how root canal procedures are performed, aiming to enhance patient care and treatment efficacy.

One of the core tenets of minimally invasive endodontics is the precision in accessing and cleaning the root canal system. Advances in endodontic microscopes and enhanced magnification techniques have revolutionized this aspect of treatment. High-powered magnification allows clinicians to visualize intricate details of the root canal anatomy that were previously obscured. This improved visualization is crucial for identifying complex canal systems, such as accessory canals and lateral canals, which are essential for effective cleaning and shaping. The use of endodontic microscopes also facilitates more precise and conservative access cavity preparations, reducing the need for extensive tooth removal and preserving healthy dentin.

In addition to magnification, the development of ultrasonic and sonic instrumentation has played a significant role in minimally invasive endodontics. Ultrasonic and sonic devices assist in the efficient cleaning and shaping of root canals with minimal mechanical intervention. These devices use high-frequency vibrations to enhance the action of irrigants and facilitate the removal of debris from the canal walls. The ability to activate irrigants effectively without aggressive file instrumentation aligns with the goal of conserving tooth structure while ensuring thorough disinfection.

Another important advancement is the refinement of root canal filling materials and techniques. Traditional root canal filling materials often required extensive preparation to ensure proper adaptation and sealing. However, contemporary bioceramic materials have emerged as a key component in minimally invasive endodontics. These materials offer excellent biocompatibility and sealing properties while requiring less aggressive shaping of the root canal. Bioceramic sealers, for instance, provide a superior seal compared to traditional gutta-percha and sealers, reducing the risk of reinfection and improving long-term outcomes.

Moreover, the approach to post-endodontic restoration has evolved to complement the minimally invasive philosophy. Post-treatment restoration strategies now prioritize the preservation of remaining tooth structure while providing adequate strength and durability. Adhesive techniques and materials, such as composite resins and glass ionomers, are employed to restore the tooth while maintaining as much of the natural tooth structure as possible. These materials bond effectively to the remaining dentin and enamel, enhancing the overall strength of the tooth and reducing the need for extensive crown preparations.

The integration of modern imaging technologies has further supported the minimally invasive approach. Cone beam computed tomography (CBCT) continues to be a valuable tool in endodontics, providing detailed three-dimensional images of the root canal system. CBCT enables clinicians to assess the complexity of the canal system, plan the treatment approach, and evaluate the success of the procedure. This level of detailed imaging supports more conservative access and shaping, as clinicians can make informed decisions based on comprehensive visual information.

Patient management and comfort are also integral to the success of minimally invasive endodontics. Advances in anesthesia techniques and materials contribute to a more comfortable experience for patients. Precise local anesthesia administration, coupled with the use of biocompatible materials, helps minimize discomfort during and after the procedure. Additionally, patient education and communication play a crucial role in managing expectations and ensuring a positive treatment experience.

The success of minimally invasive endodontics is also supported by ongoing research and clinical studies. Evidence-based practices have demonstrated that conservative approaches can yield outcomes comparable to or superior to traditional techniques, with the added benefit of preserving natural tooth structure. This body of research reinforces the importance of adopting minimally invasive methods and encourages continuous innovation in the field.

Ultimately, minimally invasive endodontics represents a significant advancement in dental care, aligning with the broader goals of preserving natural tooth structure while delivering effective and reliable treatment. By integrating advanced instruments, techniques, and materials, and focusing on patient-centered care, minimally invasive endodontics offers a forward-looking approach that enhances both clinical outcomes and patient satisfaction. The commitment to conservation and precision underscores the evolution of endodontic practice, reflecting a progressive shift towards more conservative and effective treatment methodologies.

CHAPTER 11: MINIMALLY INVASIVE PERIODONTICS

Minimally invasive periodontics represents a paradigm shift in the management of periodontal diseases, emphasizing techniques and approaches that reduce intervention severity while promoting natural tissue healing and regeneration. This chapter explores how these techniques are applied in clinical practice, with a focus on non-surgical interventions, scaling and root planing, and the use of regenerative materials.

At the heart of minimally invasive periodontics is the concept of early intervention and prevention. This approach prioritizes the identification and management of periodontal issues at their nascent stages to prevent progression to more severe forms of periodontal disease. Regular periodontal assessments and diagnostic tools, such as periodontal probing and digital imaging, are essential for detecting signs of disease early. By employing these diagnostic measures, clinicians can tailor treatments to individual needs, minimizing the extent of intervention required.

One of the foundational techniques in minimally invasive periodontics is scaling and root planing. This procedure, often referred to as deep cleaning, involves the meticulous removal of calculus and bacterial biofilm from the tooth surfaces and beneath the gum line. The goal is to create a smooth root surface that promotes the reattachment of periodontal tissues and reduces inflammation. Modern instruments and technologies, such as ultrasonic scalers, have enhanced the precision of scaling and root planing, allowing for a more thorough and comfortable treatment experience. Ultrasonic devices use high-frequency vibrations to disrupt and remove deposits from tooth surfaces with minimal discomfort to the patient, contributing to the minimally invasive philosophy.

Non-surgical periodontal therapies are complemented by a variety of adjunctive treatments aimed at improving outcomes and minimizing the need for more invasive procedures. For instance, antimicrobial agents, such as locally delivered antibiotics or antiseptic gels, can be applied directly to periodontal pockets to reduce bacterial load and inflammation. These agents work synergistically with mechanical cleaning to enhance the healing process and improve clinical outcomes.

Furthermore, the use of regenerative materials plays a pivotal role in minimally invasive periodontics. When periodontal tissue loss has occurred, regenerative techniques aim to restore lost tissue and regenerate bone. Materials such as guided tissue regeneration membranes, bone grafts, and biologic agents are employed to stimulate natural tissue regeneration. Guided tissue regeneration involves placing a barrier membrane over the defect to encourage the growth of periodontal tissues and bone while preventing the invasion of unwanted cells. Bone grafts, derived from various sources such as autogenous bone, allografts, or synthetic materials, provide a scaffold for new bone formation and support the natural healing process.

Emerging biologic agents, including growth factors and enamel matrix proteins, are also being utilized to promote periodontal tissue regeneration. These agents enhance the body's natural healing response by stimulating cell proliferation and differentiation, leading to improved tissue repair and regeneration. The application of these materials in conjunction with minimally invasive techniques underscores a shift towards biologically driven approaches in periodontal therapy.

Patient-centered care is a crucial aspect of minimally invasive periodontics. Educating patients about the importance of oral hygiene and the role of preventive measures is essential for maintaining periodontal health and preventing disease progression. Customized oral hygiene instructions, including proper brushing and flossing techniques, along with the use of adjunctive devices such as interdental brushes or water flossers, empower patients to take an active role in their periodontal care.

In addition to patient education, maintaining regular follow-up appointments is vital for monitoring periodontal health and ensuring the effectiveness of treatment. These appointments provide opportunities for ongoing evaluation, reinforcement of oral hygiene practices, and timely intervention if disease recurrence is detected. The emphasis on preventive care and early intervention aligns with the minimally invasive approach, aiming to manage periodontal conditions with minimal disruption to the patient's oral health.

The integration of technology into minimally invasive periodontics further supports the goal of precision and efficiency in periodontal care. Innovations such as digital imaging, computer-assisted diagnosis, and laser therapy enhance the accuracy of diagnostic assessments and treatment planning. Laser therapy, in particular, offers a minimally invasive alternative for various periodontal procedures, including decontamination of periodontal pockets and reduction of gingival inflammation. Lasers provide a precise and controlled approach to tissue management, reducing discomfort and promoting faster healing.

In summary, minimally invasive periodontics represents a progressive approach to managing periodontal disease with an emphasis on early intervention, non-surgical treatments, and regenerative techniques. By leveraging advancements in technology and materials, and focusing on patient-centered care, this approach aims to preserve natural tissues, enhance healing, and improve overall outcomes. The principles of minimally invasive periodontics reflect a commitment to delivering effective periodontal care while minimizing the impact on the patient's comfort and well-being.

The application of minimally invasive techniques in periodontics extends beyond traditional non-surgical interventions, integrating advanced technologies and materials to optimize treatment outcomes. As we delve further into this domain, it becomes evident that the success of minimally invasive periodontics is heavily reliant on both technological innovation and a comprehensive understanding of periodontal pathophysiology.

One of the significant advancements in minimally invasive periodontics is the use of laser technology. Lasers have revolutionized periodontal therapy by offering a precise, less invasive alternative to conventional methods. In particular, diode lasers and erbium lasers are utilized for their ability to target specific tissues with minimal damage to surrounding areas. Diode lasers are effective in managing soft tissue conditions, such as gingival hyperplasia and periodontal pocket decontamination. The laser's thermal energy helps in coagulating and sterilizing the treated area, reducing bacterial load and promoting faster healing.

Erbium lasers, on the other hand, are employed for their efficacy in both soft and hard tissue applications. They facilitate procedures such as scaling and root planing by efficiently removing calculus and necrotic tissue from the root surface while simultaneously stimulating periodontal tissue regeneration. The laser's precision allows for targeted debridement, minimizing trauma to healthy tooth structures and adjacent soft tissues.

The incorporation of technology in minimally invasive periodontics is also exemplified by advancements in diagnostic tools. The integration of digital imaging systems, such as cone beam computed tomography (CBCT), offers enhanced visualization of periodontal structures and more accurate assessment of bone levels. CBCT provides three-dimensional imaging, allowing clinicians to evaluate periodontal defects and plan interventions with greater precision. This level of detail supports better treatment planning and helps in monitoring disease progression and treatment outcomes over time.

In addition to technological advancements, the choice of materials plays a crucial role in minimally invasive periodontics. The development of novel biomaterials, including advanced regenerative agents, has significantly improved the ability to manage periodontal tissue loss and promote healing. Platelet-rich plasma (PRP) and platelet-rich fibrin (PRF) are examples of biologic materials that have gained prominence for their regenerative potential. These materials are derived from the patient's own blood and contain growth factors that facilitate tissue repair and regeneration.

PRP and PRF are utilized in various periodontal procedures, including guided tissue regeneration (GTR) and bone grafting. Their application helps in accelerating the healing process and enhancing the regeneration of periodontal tissues. The use of these biologic agents aligns with the minimally invasive philosophy by promoting natural tissue healing and minimizing the need for more invasive surgical interventions.

Another important aspect of minimally invasive periodontics is the emphasis on patient-specific treatment planning. Each patient presents unique periodontal challenges, and a tailored approach ensures that interventions are both effective and minimally disruptive. Customized treatment plans often incorporate a combination of non-surgical therapies, regenerative techniques, and patient education to address individual needs and optimize outcomes.

Patient education is a cornerstone of minimally invasive periodontics, as informed patients are more likely to engage in effective self-care and adhere to treatment recommendations. Educating patients about the nature of their periodontal condition, the rationale behind specific treatments, and the importance of maintaining good oral hygiene is essential for successful long-term management. Personalized instruction on proper brushing and flossing techniques, as well as guidance on dietary choices that impact periodontal health, empowers patients to play an active role in their treatment.

The minimally invasive approach also necessitates ongoing monitoring and maintenance to ensure the long-term success of periodontal interventions. Regular follow-up appointments are critical for evaluating the effectiveness of treatments, monitoring periodontal health, and making any necessary adjustments to the treatment plan. This proactive approach helps in identifying potential issues early and addressing them before they escalate, thereby supporting sustained periodontal health and minimizing the need for more invasive procedures.

In conclusion, the field of minimally invasive periodontics is characterized by a commitment to reducing the invasiveness of periodontal treatments while maximizing their effectiveness. The integration of advanced technologies, such as lasers and digital imaging, along with the use of innovative biomaterials and a patient-centered approach, reflects a shift towards more conservative and personalized periodontal care. By focusing on early intervention, non-surgical therapies, and patient education, minimally invasive periodontics aims to preserve natural tissues, promote healing, and enhance overall periodontal health. This approach represents a progressive step in periodontal therapy, aligning with the broader principles of minimally invasive dentistry and reinforcing the goal of achieving optimal outcomes with minimal disruption to the patient's oral health.

The effectiveness of minimally invasive periodontics relies not only on advanced techniques and materials but also on a nuanced understanding of periodontal disease and its management. As we further examine the strategies employed in this field, it becomes clear that a multi-faceted approach is essential for optimizing patient outcomes and maintaining long-term periodontal health.

One of the pivotal aspects of minimally invasive periodontics is the precise execution of scaling and root planing (SRP). This foundational non-surgical procedure aims to remove bacterial plaque and calculus from tooth surfaces and root areas, thereby reducing inflammation and promoting periodontal tissue healing. The technique involves meticulous cleaning of the tooth surfaces, including the subgingival areas, which are often challenging to access. The advent of ultrasonic scaling devices has enhanced the effectiveness of SRP by providing efficient and gentle removal of deposits. These instruments use high-frequency vibrations to dislodge calculus and biofilm, minimizing tissue damage and improving patient comfort.

Following SRP, the management of periodontal pockets and the promotion of tissue regeneration become crucial. Traditional methods often involve the use of local antibiotics or antimicrobial agents to further reduce bacterial load and prevent infection. In recent years, the application of advanced regenerative materials has transformed this aspect of treatment. Materials such as collagen membranes and bioactive glass have been introduced to support periodontal tissue regeneration. Collagen membranes serve as a scaffold for new tissue growth, aiding in the healing of bone and soft tissue defects. Bioactive glass, with its ability to bond with bone and stimulate mineralization, has been used to enhance the repair of periodontal bone loss.

The concept of guided tissue regeneration (GTR) represents a significant advancement in minimally invasive periodontics. GTR involves the use of barrier membranes to direct the growth of periodontal tissues while excluding non-periodontal tissues from the regenerative site. This approach not only promotes the healing of bone and soft tissues but also prevents the invasion of unwanted tissues into the treatment area. The selection of appropriate membranes and regenerative materials is based on a thorough assessment of the patient's specific needs and the nature of the periodontal defect.

Another critical component of minimally invasive periodontics is the focus on preventing disease recurrence through proactive maintenance and monitoring. After initial therapy, patients are typically placed on a structured maintenance program that includes regular periodontal check-ups and professional cleanings. This preventive approach is essential for managing periodontal disease over the long term and preventing the progression of any remaining disease. The frequency of maintenance visits is determined based on individual risk factors, including the severity of the initial disease and the patient's overall health and compliance.

Patient education remains a cornerstone of effective periodontal management. Empowering patients with knowledge about the nature of their condition and the importance of maintaining oral hygiene can significantly impact treatment outcomes. This involves not only instructing patients on proper brushing and flossing techniques but also discussing lifestyle factors that may influence periodontal health. For instance, patients who smoke are at a higher risk of periodontal disease progression, and cessation counseling becomes an integral part of the treatment plan.

Additionally, the role of diet in periodontal health cannot be overlooked. Nutritional counseling, which emphasizes a balanced diet rich in vitamins and minerals, supports immune function and tissue repair. Patients are encouraged to incorporate foods that promote oral health and avoid those that may exacerbate periodontal issues.

The integration of technology in monitoring and managing periodontal health also plays a vital role in minimally invasive practices. The use of electronic health records and digital imaging systems facilitates comprehensive tracking of treatment progress and patient outcomes. These tools enable clinicians to make data-driven decisions and adjust treatment plans as necessary based on real-time feedback.

In conclusion, minimally invasive periodontics encompasses a range of techniques and approaches designed to manage periodontal disease with the least amount of intervention required. From advanced scaling and root planing methods to the use of regenerative materials and barrier membranes, the field has evolved to emphasize tissue preservation and patient-centered care. The combination of non-surgical interventions, patient education, and ongoing maintenance reflects a commitment to preserving natural tooth structures and promoting long-term periodontal health. By embracing these principles, dental professionals can achieve successful outcomes while adhering to the core tenets of minimally invasive dentistry.

CHAPTER 12: MINIMALLY INVASIVE ORTHODONTICS

The field of orthodontics has experienced significant advancements in recent years, particularly with the adoption of minimally invasive techniques. These innovations aim to achieve effective orthodontic outcomes while minimizing the impact on oral health and patient comfort. This chapter delves into the contemporary approaches in minimally invasive orthodontics, exploring the application of clear aligners, minimally invasive brackets, and other technologies that represent a departure from traditional, more invasive methods.

Clear aligners have revolutionized orthodontic treatment by offering a more aesthetic and comfortable alternative to conventional braces. These removable appliances are custom-made to fit the patient's teeth and are designed to gradually shift them into their desired positions. The primary advantage of clear aligners is their ability to achieve tooth movement without the need for metal brackets and wires, which often cause discomfort and require frequent adjustments. Aligners are made from a smooth, transparent plastic, which enhances patient comfort and reduces the risk of oral irritation. Additionally, their removable nature allows for easier oral hygiene maintenance, as patients can take them out to brush and floss, thus preventing plaque accumulation and the potential for dental caries.

The efficacy of clear aligners is largely attributed to advancements in digital orthodontics. Computer-aided design (CAD) and computer-aided manufacturing (CAM) technologies play a critical role in the creation of these aligners. Through 3D imaging and modeling, orthodontists can precisely plan the sequence of tooth movements required for treatment. This digital approach not only enhances the accuracy of aligner fabrication but also allows for the simulation of treatment outcomes before the actual appliances are manufactured. As a result, patients can visualize their expected results, which can improve their adherence to the treatment plan.

Minimally invasive brackets represent another significant advancement in orthodontic technology. Unlike traditional metal brackets, which are often bulky and require extensive enamel reduction for bonding, minimally invasive brackets are designed to be smaller and less obtrusive. These brackets use advanced adhesive systems that require less enamel preparation, thereby preserving more of the tooth's natural structure. The reduced size and weight of these brackets also contribute to greater patient comfort and less noticeable orthodontic appliances.

Furthermore, the development of self-ligating brackets has added another layer of innovation to minimally invasive orthodontics. Self-ligating brackets utilize a built-in mechanism to hold the archwire in place, eliminating the need for elastic or metal ligatures. This design reduces friction between the bracket and wire, which can lead to more efficient tooth movement and less discomfort during treatment. Additionally, self-ligating brackets often require fewer adjustments compared to traditional brackets, which can shorten overall treatment time and reduce the frequency of office visits.

Another noteworthy advancement in minimally invasive orthodontics is the use of temporary anchorage devices (TADs). TADs are small, screw-like implants that provide a stable anchor point for certain orthodontic movements, particularly those that involve significant tooth repositioning. These devices are minimally invasive and can be placed with a simple surgical procedure that typically requires only local anesthesia. TADs enable orthodontists to achieve complex tooth movements that would otherwise be difficult or impossible with traditional methods, all while minimizing the need for more invasive procedures such as extraction or jaw surgery.

The application of digital tools and techniques extends beyond the planning and execution of orthodontic treatment. Innovations in 3D imaging, such as cone beam computed tomography (CBCT), allow for a detailed assessment of the dental and skeletal structures. This advanced imaging technique provides comprehensive information about the tooth roots, bone density, and spatial relationships, which can significantly enhance the precision of orthodontic diagnosis and treatment planning. By integrating these digital tools, orthodontists can better tailor their interventions to each patient's unique anatomy and needs.

Patient education is a crucial component of successful minimally invasive orthodontic treatment. Educating patients about the benefits and limitations of different orthodontic options empowers them to make informed decisions about their care. Clear communication regarding the expected outcomes, treatment duration, and maintenance requirements helps manage patient expectations and promotes adherence to the treatment plan.

In summary, the landscape of orthodontics is increasingly shaped by minimally invasive techniques that prioritize patient comfort, oral health, and effective outcomes. The advent of clear aligners, minimally invasive brackets, and innovative devices like TADs exemplifies the shift towards more conservative and patient-friendly orthodontic care. By leveraging these advancements, orthodontists can provide high-quality treatment while minimizing the impact on the patient's oral health and overall well-being. The continued evolution of these technologies promises to further enhance the field, offering even more refined and effective solutions for achieving optimal orthodontic results.

In the realm of minimally invasive orthodontics, the integration of advanced technologies and materials continues to redefine patient care by emphasizing less intrusive methods. This shift is primarily driven by the desire to enhance patient comfort while achieving optimal orthodontic results. As previously explored, clear aligners and minimally invasive brackets have set a new standard in orthodontic practice. However, additional technologies and approaches further illustrate the evolution of this field and its commitment to minimizing patient discomfort and oral health impacts.

One of the prominent advancements in minimally invasive orthodontics is the use of accelerated orthodontic techniques. These methods, designed to expedite the movement of teeth, complement traditional and modern orthodontic appliances by reducing the overall treatment duration. Techniques such as Propel and AcceleDent use micro-osteoperforation or vibrational forces to stimulate bone remodeling and accelerate tooth movement. These interventions are minimally invasive, typically involving only small incisions or vibrational devices that the patient uses at home. By shortening treatment times, these techniques not only improve patient satisfaction but also decrease the overall period of appliance wear, further aligning with minimally invasive principles.

Another significant development is the use of digital orthodontic platforms that enhance treatment planning and monitoring. Digital workflow tools, including intraoral scanners and 3D imaging systems, enable orthodontists to create highly accurate digital models of patients' dentition. These models facilitate precise treatment planning and allow for real-time adjustments to be made as treatment progresses. The increased accuracy provided by these digital tools helps in minimizing the need for manual adjustments, thereby reducing the frequency of patient visits and the associated discomfort.

3D printing technology has also emerged as a transformative force in minimally invasive orthodontics. This technology allows for the rapid production of customized orthodontic appliances, such as retainers and aligners, with high precision. The use of 3D printing enables orthodontists to provide patients with appliances that fit more comfortably and function more effectively than those produced using traditional methods. Additionally, the ability to quickly produce and modify appliances based on real-time feedback from digital scans contributes to a more efficient and patient-friendly treatment process.

The role of patient-specific customization has been greatly enhanced through these technological advancements. Custom orthodontic appliances, including clear aligners and brackets, can now be designed and fabricated to precisely match each patient's unique dental anatomy. This level of customization ensures that the appliances are more effective in achieving the desired tooth movements while minimizing any discomfort or issues associated with ill-fitting devices.

In addition to technological innovations, the focus on preventive orthodontics represents a growing trend within the field. Preventive orthodontics involves the early intervention and management of potential orthodontic issues before they require more invasive treatment. This approach includes the use of interceptive orthodontic techniques, which aim to correct malocclusions and other dental issues during the mixed dentition phase. By addressing these concerns early, orthodontists can often avoid the need for more extensive interventions later in life, aligning with the principles of minimally invasive care.

Furthermore, the emphasis on patient education and engagement plays a crucial role in minimally invasive orthodontics. Educating patients about the benefits and limitations of different orthodontic options, as well as providing guidance on maintaining oral hygiene and adhering to treatment protocols, can significantly impact the success of minimally invasive treatments. Empowered with knowledge, patients are more likely to actively participate in their treatment and follow the prescribed care regimen, which contributes to better outcomes and reduced need for corrective measures.

As the field of orthodontics continues to evolve, the integration of minimally invasive techniques remains central to enhancing patient care. The advancements in clear aligners, minimally invasive brackets, accelerated orthodontic techniques, digital tools, and 3D printing underscore the commitment to achieving effective orthodontic outcomes with minimal impact on oral health. These innovations reflect a broader trend towards more conservative and patient-centered approaches in orthodontics, aiming to improve both the efficacy of treatment and the overall patient experience. As research and technology progress, further refinements in minimally invasive orthodontics are anticipated, promising even more sophisticated and patient-friendly solutions for achieving optimal dental alignment and function.

The paradigm shift toward minimally invasive orthodontics

reflects a broader commitment to enhancing patient comfort and streamlining orthodontic care. This shift is facilitated not only by advances in technology but also by a deeper understanding of the biological processes involved in tooth movement and the ways in which treatment protocols can be optimized.

A key component of minimally invasive orthodontics is the refinement of bracket and wire systems. Traditional fixed appliances have evolved significantly, and contemporary brackets are designed with patient comfort as a priority. Modern brackets are often smaller and more streamlined, reducing the discomfort and irritation commonly associated with earlier models. Innovations in bracket design, such as those incorporating self-ligating mechanisms, further minimize the need for frequent adjustments and reduce the overall force exerted on the teeth. These systems use specialized clips or doors to hold the wire in place, decreasing friction and making adjustments less cumbersome for both the patient and the clinician.

Another advancement in minimally invasive orthodontics is the development of personalized treatment plans through advanced digital technologies. The use of digital treatment planning software allows orthodontists to simulate the movement of teeth and predict outcomes with a high degree of accuracy. These simulations enable orthodontists to tailor treatment plans to each patient's specific needs, reducing the likelihood of unexpected complications and the need for extensive adjustments. By visualizing the end result before beginning treatment, orthodontists can make more informed decisions, leading to more efficient and less invasive procedures.

Clear aligners, which have become a cornerstone of minimally invasive orthodontics, represent a significant departure from traditional metal braces. These aligners are custom-made to fit each patient's dentition precisely, applying gentle, consistent pressure to move teeth into their desired positions. The aligners are made from transparent, flexible materials that are both comfortable and less noticeable than traditional braces. The removable nature of aligners also allows patients to maintain better oral hygiene, as they can brush and floss without the obstruction of fixed appliances. This feature helps in reducing the risk of secondary issues such as enamel demineralization and gingival irritation.

The technology behind clear aligners continues to advance, with new materials and manufacturing techniques improving their effectiveness and comfort. Innovations such as 3D-printed aligners and advanced thermoplastic materials enhance the durability and precision of the aligners, leading to more predictable and efficient treatment outcomes. Additionally, the integration of artificial intelligence into aligner design and treatment planning processes helps in predicting tooth movements and optimizing aligner adjustments.

In conjunction with clear aligners, minimally invasive orthodontics also benefits from the use of adjunctive therapies that support and accelerate tooth movement. For instance, devices that apply microvibrations or gentle pulsations to the teeth and surrounding tissues can stimulate bone remodeling and accelerate the orthodontic process. These adjunctive treatments are minimally invasive and often involve devices that can be used at home, further enhancing patient convenience and comfort.

Moreover, the concept of minimally invasive orthodontics extends to the management of orthodontic relapse and retention. Retainers, which are critical for maintaining tooth positions post-treatment, are now available in more comfortable and less obtrusive forms. The evolution of retainer materials and designs, such as vacuum-formed retainers, aligns with the principles of minimally invasive care by providing effective retention without compromising patient comfort.

The integration of minimally invasive orthodontics also involves a focus on preventive care and early intervention. By identifying and addressing potential orthodontic issues early in a patient's development, orthodontists can often avoid more invasive treatments later. Early intervention strategies include the use of interceptive appliances that address issues such as overcrowding or crossbites before they require more extensive intervention. This proactive approach not only aligns with minimally invasive principles but also enhances the overall effectiveness of orthodontic care.

The future of minimally invasive orthodontics promises continued innovation and refinement. Ongoing research into new materials, technologies, and techniques aims to further enhance the efficacy and comfort of orthodontic treatments. As the field evolves, the emphasis will likely remain on developing solutions that maximize patient comfort, minimize intervention, and achieve optimal outcomes with the least disruption to oral health.

In summary, the practice of minimally invasive orthodontics embodies a commitment to enhancing patient care through technological innovation and refined techniques. By leveraging advances in digital technology, personalized treatment plans, and non-invasive adjunctive therapies, orthodontists can offer effective treatment while minimizing patient discomfort and preserving oral health. As these approaches continue to evolve, they promise to further transform the landscape of orthodontic care, making it more patient-centered and less intrusive.

CHAPTER 13: DIGITAL INTEGRATION IN MINIMALLY INVASIVE DENTISTRY

The integration of digital technologies into minimally invasive dentistry represents a transformative shift in the field, characterized by enhancements in precision, efficiency, and patient comfort. This chapter delves into the various digital tools and systems that are revolutionizing dental practice, particularly focusing on how these innovations align with the principles of minimally invasive treatment.

One of the most significant advancements in digital integration is the use of digital impressions. Traditional methods of obtaining dental impressions, which involved the use of impression trays and materials that could be uncomfortable and often resulted in inaccuracies, are being increasingly supplanted by digital impression systems. These systems utilize intraoral scanners to capture high-resolution, three-dimensional images of the teeth and oral tissues. The accuracy of digital impressions surpasses that of conventional methods, reducing the need for retakes and minimizing patient discomfort. By providing precise and immediate results, digital impressions facilitate the creation of restorations that fit more accurately and comfortably, enhancing the overall outcome of minimally invasive procedures.

Complementing digital impressions are CAD/CAM (Computer-Aided Design and Computer-Aided Manufacturing) systems. CAD/CAM technology allows for the design and production of dental restorations, such as crowns, bridges, and inlays, directly from digital scans. The CAD component involves designing the restoration on a computer using specialized software that translates the digital impression into a detailed model. The CAM component then uses this design to manufacture the restoration using milling machines or 3D printers. This process streamlines the workflow by enabling the creation of custom restorations with high precision and speed. Additionally, CAD/CAM technology reduces the number of visits required for patients, as restorations can often be completed in a single appointment, aligning with the minimally invasive principle of reducing treatment duration and improving patient convenience.

The benefits of digital integration extend beyond the creation of restorations. Digital radiography and imaging systems offer significant advantages over traditional radiographic techniques. Digital sensors provide high-resolution images with reduced radiation exposure, enabling more accurate diagnosis and treatment planning. The ability to enhance and manipulate digital images in real time facilitates a more thorough assessment of the patient's condition and supports the development of targeted, minimally invasive treatment plans. Digital imaging also allows for easy sharing and collaboration among dental professionals, enhancing the coordination of care and improving treatment outcomes.

Another notable advancement is the use of digital treatment planning software, which integrates with CAD/CAM systems and digital imaging tools. This software enables orthodontists and other dental specialists to create detailed, three-dimensional treatment plans based on digital models of the patient's dentition. By simulating various treatment scenarios, dental professionals can predict outcomes with greater accuracy and tailor treatment plans to each patient's unique needs. This level of precision supports minimally invasive approaches by optimizing the use of conservative techniques and minimizing the need for extensive adjustments or alterations during treatment.

The incorporation of digital workflows also enhances the ability to perform minimally invasive procedures with greater precision. For example, guided surgery systems, which utilize digital imaging and planning software to create surgical guides, enable more accurate placement of implants or other interventions. These guides ensure that procedures are performed with minimal disruption to surrounding tissues and structures, aligning with the minimally invasive ethos of preserving as much natural tissue as possible.

Furthermore, digital tools facilitate patient education and engagement. Digital simulations and visualizations allow patients to see potential outcomes before undergoing treatment, improving their understanding and expectations of the procedures. This not only enhances patient satisfaction but also helps in gaining informed consent by providing a clearer picture of the anticipated results.

The ongoing evolution of digital technologies in dentistry continues to open new possibilities for enhancing minimally invasive practices. Innovations such as artificial intelligence and machine learning are beginning to play a role in analyzing digital data, predicting treatment outcomes, and personalizing care. These advancements promise to further refine the precision and effectiveness of minimally invasive techniques, making dental procedures less invasive and more tailored to individual patient needs.

In conclusion, the integration of digital technologies into minimally invasive dentistry represents a significant advancement in the field. By improving the accuracy of diagnostics, streamlining the creation of restorations, and enhancing the overall patient experience, digital tools align with the principles of minimally invasive care. As these technologies continue to evolve, they will undoubtedly contribute to further advancements in dental practice, making treatments more efficient, precise, and comfortable for patients while adhering to the core tenets of minimally invasive dentistry.

The evolution of digital technologies has introduced transformative changes in minimally invasive dentistry, enhancing precision, efficiency, and patient comfort through various innovative tools. Building on the foundation of digital impressions and CAD/CAM systems, several other technological advancements contribute to refining minimally invasive practices.

Digital workflows in endodontics, for instance, illustrate how digital tools facilitate minimally invasive treatments. Endodontic procedures, traditionally characterized by their complexity and potential for extensive tooth preparation, benefit significantly from digital integration. Digital apex locators, which provide real-time measurements of root canal length, enhance the accuracy of root canal treatments. By minimizing the need for manual measurements and reducing the risk of over-instrumentation, these tools support more conservative endodontic procedures.

Furthermore, advancements in cone beam computed tomography (CBCT) have revolutionized diagnostic imaging in endodontics and other areas of dentistry. CBCT provides three-dimensional imaging of the teeth, bones, and surrounding structures, allowing for a comprehensive assessment of complex cases with minimal radiation exposure compared to conventional computed tomography. This detailed imaging capability supports more precise planning for minimally invasive procedures, such as endodontic treatments and implant placements, by offering a clear view of the root canal system and anatomical variations that might impact treatment.

In orthodontics, digital technologies have also led to the development of less invasive treatment modalities. Clear aligners, for instance, are a prime example of how digital integration enhances orthodontic care. Digital scans of the patient's dentition create a precise 3D model, which is used to design a series of custom aligners. This approach not only avoids the need for traditional metal brackets and wires but also allows for more predictable and gradual tooth movement. The ability to visualize the treatment outcome before initiating therapy helps in planning a minimally invasive approach that addresses alignment issues without compromising oral health.

The use of digital tools extends to the realm of prosthodontics as well. The integration of digital systems into prosthetic planning and fabrication enables the design and production of highly accurate restorations. For example, digital bite registration and occlusal analysis tools provide precise data on the patient's occlusion, which is critical for creating well-fitting crowns, bridges, and dentures. By utilizing these digital tools, prosthodontists can achieve optimal fit and function with minimal adjustment, aligning with the principles of minimally invasive dentistry.

Digital integration also enhances patient engagement and education. Advanced visualization tools, such as digital smile design software, enable patients to see simulated results of proposed treatments, including cosmetic and functional changes. This interactive approach allows patients to make informed decisions and contributes to a more collaborative treatment planning process. By incorporating patient preferences and expectations into the digital planning, dental professionals can tailor minimally invasive treatments to better meet individual needs.

The role of artificial intelligence (AI) in digital dentistry is emerging as a significant advancement with implications for minimally invasive procedures. AI algorithms can analyze large datasets from digital images, helping to identify patterns and anomalies that might be missed by the human eye. In diagnostic applications, AI can assist in detecting early signs of carious lesions, periodontal disease, or other conditions, facilitating earlier intervention and more conservative management. Additionally, AI-driven tools can optimize treatment planning by predicting outcomes based on historical data and patient-specific variables.

As digital technologies continue to advance, their integration into minimally invasive dentistry is expected to become even more profound. Innovations such as real-time intraoral sensors and advanced materials for 3D printing are likely to further enhance the precision and efficiency of dental procedures. The ongoing development of digital platforms that integrate seamlessly with existing dental technologies will contribute to a more cohesive and streamlined approach to patient care.

In summary, the integration of digital technologies in minimally invasive dentistry has brought about significant improvements in precision, efficiency, and patient comfort. Digital impressions, CAD/CAM systems, and other advanced tools have transformed various aspects of dental practice, from diagnostic imaging to treatment planning and patient engagement. As these technologies continue to evolve, they will further refine minimally invasive approaches, making dental care more precise, efficient, and patient-centered. The ongoing advancement of digital tools promises to support the goals of minimally invasive dentistry, providing enhanced outcomes while preserving as much natural tooth structure as possible.

The integration of digital technologies in minimally invasive dentistry has not only streamlined procedures but also set new standards in patient care and clinical outcomes. These advancements are reshaping how dental practices approach treatment planning, execution, and follow-up, contributing significantly to the evolution of minimally invasive techniques.

One of the most notable contributions of digital technology is the enhancement of diagnostic accuracy. Digital radiography, for instance, offers a significant improvement over traditional film-based methods. By providing instant image capture and the ability to manipulate the images digitally, clinicians can more accurately assess dental conditions. Digital radiographs also reduce the radiation exposure to patients, aligning with the minimally invasive ethos of reducing harm while maintaining diagnostic efficacy. The high-resolution images allow for detailed examination of tooth structures and surrounding tissues, facilitating early detection and intervention of carious lesions, periodontal issues, and other abnormalities with minimal disruption to the patient.

In conjunction with digital radiography, the use of intraoral cameras has revolutionized how dental conditions are visualized and communicated. Intraoral cameras capture high-quality images of the oral cavity, allowing both clinicians and patients to see real-time views of their dental health. This visual feedback is invaluable for patient education, as it helps patients understand the necessity of proposed treatments and the benefits of maintaining oral health. The integration of these images into digital records enhances the continuity of care, as clinicians can track changes over time and adjust treatment plans accordingly.

The application of CAD/CAM (Computer-Aided Design/Computer-Aided Manufacturing) technology represents a significant leap forward in the fabrication of dental restorations. CAD/CAM systems enable the precise design and manufacturing of crowns, bridges, inlays, and onlays with a high degree of accuracy. The process begins with digital impressions, which are captured using intraoral scanners. These digital impressions eliminate the need for traditional, often uncomfortable, physical impressions and provide a more accurate representation of the tooth's structure. The digital models are then used to design restorations that fit seamlessly with the patient's existing dental anatomy. CAD/CAM technology streamlines the production process, reducing the number of patient visits required and improving the overall efficiency of restorative procedures.

Another important aspect of digital integration is the use of virtual treatment planning in orthodontics. Clear aligner therapy, supported by digital modeling and simulation, has transformed orthodontic treatment. Patients receive a customized treatment plan based on 3D digital scans of their dentition, which allows for the creation of a series of aligners that incrementally move the teeth into the desired positions. This technology not only improves the predictability of treatment outcomes but also enhances patient comfort and compliance by reducing the need for traditional metal brackets and wires. Virtual planning tools also enable clinicians to visualize the final treatment result before starting therapy, ensuring that the treatment plan aligns with the patient's goals and expectations.

Digital integration extends beyond diagnostics and treatment planning to include advanced materials and fabrication techniques. The use of 3D printing in dentistry is a prime example of how digital technology can support minimally invasive approaches. 3D printing enables the rapid production of dental models, surgical guides, and even prosthetic components. This technology allows for precise customization and quick turnaround times, contributing to more efficient and less invasive procedures. For instance, 3D-printed surgical guides can assist in the accurate placement of dental implants, reducing the need for extensive flap surgery and enhancing the precision of implant placement.

Moreover, the integration of digital workflows into dental practices enhances patient comfort and reduces clinical chair time. Automated systems for tasks such as digital charting, appointment scheduling, and treatment planning streamline administrative processes, allowing clinicians to focus more on patient care. These systems also facilitate better communication between the dental team and the patient, improving overall treatment experience and outcomes.

Looking ahead, the continued advancement of digital technologies promises even greater innovations in minimally invasive dentistry. Emerging technologies such as augmented reality (AR) and artificial intelligence (AI) are poised to further refine treatment approaches. AR can assist clinicians in visualizing complex procedures in real time, providing a layer of guidance during minimally invasive surgeries. AI has the potential to analyze vast amounts of dental data to predict treatment outcomes, optimize procedures, and personalize patient care.

In conclusion, the integration of digital technologies into minimally invasive dentistry has transformed the field by enhancing diagnostic accuracy, improving treatment planning, and increasing patient comfort. The continuous development of digital tools and techniques supports the goals of minimally invasive dentistry by providing precise, efficient, and patient-centered care. As these technologies evolve, they will undoubtedly lead to further advancements in dental practice, reinforcing the commitment to preserving natural tooth structure and optimizing oral health outcomes.

CHAPTER 14: FUTURE TRENDS IN MINIMALLY INVASIVE DENTISTRY

As the field of minimally invasive dentistry progresses, emerging technologies and innovative materials promise to redefine the boundaries of dental practice. This chapter explores the anticipated advancements that are likely to influence the evolution of minimally invasive techniques, further improving patient care and enhancing clinical outcomes.

The future of minimally invasive dentistry is closely intertwined with the ongoing development of digital technologies. One of the most promising areas is the integration of artificial intelligence (AI) into diagnostic and treatment planning processes. AI algorithms, trained on vast datasets of dental images and patient records, have the potential to enhance diagnostic accuracy and predict treatment outcomes with unprecedented precision. By analyzing patterns and anomalies in dental imagery, AI can assist clinicians in identifying early signs of carious lesions, periodontal disease, and other conditions that may not be readily apparent through traditional diagnostic methods. This capability will enable earlier interventions and more tailored treatment plans, aligning perfectly with the principles of minimally invasive dentistry.

Another significant advancement on the horizon is the continued evolution of 3D printing technology. While 3D printing has already made substantial contributions to restorative dentistry through the creation of custom prosthetics and surgical guides, future developments are expected to further expand its applications. Innovations in 3D printing materials and techniques will likely lead to the production of even more precise and biocompatible dental restorations. Additionally, the ability to print complex structures at a micro-scale could revolutionize the creation of dental implants and orthodontic appliances, making them more adaptable and less invasive.

The integration of regenerative medicine into minimally invasive dentistry is another area of exciting potential. Advances in stem cell research and tissue engineering may soon provide new ways to repair and regenerate damaged tooth structures and periodontal tissues. Techniques such as the use of bioactive materials that promote tissue regeneration and the application of growth factors to stimulate natural healing processes are expected to become more refined and widely adopted. These approaches hold the promise of not only repairing damaged tissues with minimal intervention but also potentially reversing some of the damage associated with dental conditions.

The development of novel biomaterials is also anticipated to play a crucial role in shaping the future of minimally invasive dentistry. Researchers are continually exploring new materials that offer superior strength, aesthetics, and biocompatibility. For instance, the advent of advanced composite resins and glass ionomer materials with enhanced properties will enable more effective and durable restorations while preserving more of the natural tooth structure. Additionally, materials that actively contribute to the prevention of caries and other dental issues through antimicrobial or remineralizing effects are likely to become integral to minimally invasive practices.

Minimally invasive orthodontics is poised for transformation with the ongoing advancements in clear aligner technology. Future developments in aligner materials and digital planning tools will likely lead to even greater customization and precision in orthodontic treatment. Enhanced software algorithms and AI integration will enable orthodontists to simulate treatment outcomes with greater accuracy, resulting in more efficient and effective alignment processes. Moreover, innovations in appliance design and material science may lead to more comfortable and less obtrusive orthodontic solutions.

The role of tele-dentistry is also expected to expand significantly. As remote consultation technologies become more sophisticated, they will facilitate more widespread access to dental care, particularly for patients in underserved or remote areas. Tele-dentistry will enable real-time consultations, remote monitoring of treatment progress, and virtual follow-up care, all of which align with the principles of minimally invasive dentistry by reducing the need for physical interventions and enhancing patient convenience.

Additionally, the concept of personalized dentistry is likely to gain momentum. Advances in genomics and personalized medicine will allow for a more tailored approach to dental care, where treatment plans are customized based on an individual's genetic predispositions and unique oral health needs. This personalization will contribute to more effective and targeted minimally invasive treatments, enhancing both patient outcomes and satisfaction.

Finally, as minimally invasive dentistry continues to evolve, there will be an increased emphasis on interdisciplinary approaches to patient care. Collaboration between dental specialists, general practitioners, and other healthcare providers will become more integrated, ensuring a comprehensive approach to managing oral health that considers the broader context of overall health and well-being.

In conclusion, the future of minimally invasive dentistry is marked by rapid technological advancements, innovative materials, and evolving techniques that promise to further enhance patient care. The integration of AI, 3D printing, regenerative medicine, and personalized approaches will drive the next generation of minimally invasive practices, making dental treatments more precise, effective, and patient-centered. As these trends unfold, they will reinforce the core principles of minimally invasive dentistry—preserving natural tooth structure, minimizing patient discomfort, and improving overall outcomes. The ongoing commitment to innovation and excellence will ensure that minimally invasive dentistry continues to advance and adapt to meet the evolving needs of patients and the field.

As we look ahead in minimally invasive dentistry, the integration of emerging technologies and materials will continue to refine the field, offering new opportunities for more effective, patient-centered care. One of the most transformative developments in this domain is the advancement of real-time diagnostic imaging and monitoring technologies. These innovations include intraoral cameras, advanced radiographic systems, and optical coherence tomography (OCT), all of which enable clinicians to capture highly detailed images of the oral cavity with minimal discomfort to the patient. These tools not only improve diagnostic accuracy but also enhance the ability to monitor the progression of dental conditions with greater precision, allowing for more timely and conservative interventions.

In particular, OCT, a non-invasive imaging technique that

provides cross-sectional images of tissues, has shown promise in detecting early carious lesions and assessing the depth of decay without the need for traditional radiography. By allowing clinicians to visualize subsurface dental structures in detail, OCT supports the minimally invasive approach by enabling earlier detection of problems and thereby reducing the extent of treatment needed.

Another area of significant advancement is in the development of bioactive materials, which represent a paradigm shift in restorative dentistry. Unlike traditional materials, bioactive materials are designed to interact with biological tissues to promote healing and regeneration. For example, calcium phosphate-based materials and bioactive glass can release ions that stimulate the formation of new, healthy tooth structure or enhance the remineralization of early carious lesions. These materials offer the dual benefit of repairing damaged teeth while simultaneously encouraging natural repair processes, thereby aligning with the minimally invasive philosophy of preserving as much healthy tissue as possible.

Additionally, the field of regenerative dentistry is experiencing rapid growth. Techniques such as tissue engineering and stem cell therapy are being explored to address dental issues with minimal intervention. Research into stem cells derived from dental pulp or periodontal tissues may soon provide methods for regenerating lost tooth structure or even whole teeth. Such advances hold the potential to transform the treatment of severe dental conditions, allowing for more natural restoration of oral function and aesthetics.

The use of personalized treatment plans driven by genetic information is also on the horizon. By incorporating genetic and epigenetic data, dental professionals can tailor treatments to the individual patient's specific needs and predispositions. This approach not only enhances the effectiveness of preventive and restorative procedures but also minimizes the risk of adverse outcomes. Personalized dentistry promises to make treatments more efficient and effective, reducing the need for more invasive procedures by addressing issues at their root cause.

In parallel with these technological and material innovations, the trend toward more sophisticated patient management strategies is gaining momentum. The implementation of patient-specific digital records and enhanced data analytics will facilitate a more comprehensive approach to oral health management. Digital tools will enable better tracking of treatment progress, personalized follow-up care, and the ability to anticipate and address potential issues before they require more invasive interventions.

Moreover, the rise of tele-dentistry will likely continue to expand, providing more accessible care options for patients who may have difficulties accessing traditional dental services. Remote consultations, virtual diagnostics, and digital treatment planning are expected to become more prevalent, offering patients the convenience of receiving expert care without the need for frequent in-office visits. This shift towards tele-dentistry supports the minimally invasive philosophy by reducing the need for physical interventions and allowing for more flexible and personalized care.

Educational advancements are also anticipated to play a crucial role in shaping the future of minimally invasive dentistry. As new techniques and technologies emerge, dental education and training will evolve to ensure that practitioners are well-versed in the latest advancements. Continued emphasis on evidence-based practice and interdisciplinary collaboration will enhance the integration of minimally invasive methods into everyday dental practice.

In summary, the future of minimally invasive dentistry

is marked by rapid technological advancements, innovative materials, and evolving treatment strategies. Real-time diagnostic imaging, bioactive materials, regenerative techniques, personalized treatments, and tele-dentistry are all set to redefine the landscape of dental care. These developments will not only improve the precision and effectiveness of minimally invasive procedures but also enhance patient comfort and outcomes. As the field progresses, the commitment to preserving natural tooth structure and minimizing patient discomfort will remain at the core of practice, driven by the ongoing pursuit of excellence and innovation.

As we advance into the future of minimally invasive dentistry, the convergence of emerging technologies and evolving techniques will further refine and elevate the practice. The focus on preserving natural tooth structure and enhancing patient comfort is set to become more sophisticated with the integration of several key innovations.

One of the most promising areas is the development of advanced biomaterials with enhanced properties. Current research is exploring materials that not only mimic the mechanical properties of natural tooth structure but also offer dynamic interaction with biological tissues. For instance, smart biomaterials that respond to environmental changes within the oral cavity could become pivotal in the management of dental issues. These materials might release therapeutic agents in response to bacterial presence or changes in pH, actively contributing to the prevention and treatment of carious lesions and other dental conditions.

The future of minimally invasive dentistry will also likely be influenced by advancements in nanotechnology. Nanomaterials, with their unique properties and ability to interact at the molecular level, hold significant potential for improving dental treatments. Nanocomposites, for example, can provide enhanced mechanical properties and better aesthetic outcomes. Additionally, nanoparticles could be used for targeted drug delivery, allowing for localized treatment of dental diseases and promoting faster healing with minimal intervention.

Another trend that is anticipated to gain momentum is the use of artificial intelligence (AI) and machine learning in diagnostic and treatment planning processes. AI algorithms can analyze vast amounts of patient data, including digital impressions and radiographic images, to assist in diagnosing dental conditions with higher accuracy. Machine learning models can predict the progression of dental diseases and recommend personalized treatment plans based on a patient's unique characteristics and historical data. This approach promises not only to enhance diagnostic precision but also to facilitate more effective and minimally invasive interventions.

Digital workflows and automation are also poised to revolutionize minimally invasive dentistry. The integration of robotic systems into dental practices could lead to more precise and controlled procedures. For instance, robotic-assisted techniques might improve the accuracy of placing restorations or performing delicate surgical procedures, reducing the need for extensive tooth preparation and minimizing patient discomfort. Additionally, automated systems for fabricating dental prosthetics and restorations can enhance the speed and accuracy of these processes, further aligning with the principles of minimally invasive care.

The expansion of regenerative dentistry will play a crucial role in the future landscape of minimally invasive techniques. Stem cell research and tissue engineering are rapidly evolving, offering the potential to regenerate damaged tooth structures and periodontal tissues. Innovations in scaffolding materials and cell-based therapies might one day allow for the complete regeneration of lost dental structures, reducing the need for more invasive restorative procedures and promoting natural healing processes.

Tele-dentistry and remote monitoring will continue to transform patient management and care delivery. The use of telehealth platforms for virtual consultations and follow-ups will become increasingly prevalent, providing patients with convenient access to dental care while minimizing the need for in-office visits. Remote monitoring technologies, including wearable devices that track oral health metrics, can offer real-time data to both patients and clinicians, allowing for proactive management of dental conditions and timely intervention when necessary.

Educational advancements will also shape the future of minimally invasive dentistry. The integration of virtual reality (VR) and augmented reality (AR) into dental education and training can provide immersive learning experiences, enabling students and practitioners to practice and refine their skills in a simulated environment. These technologies can enhance understanding of complex procedures and improve clinical outcomes by allowing for hands-on practice without the risk of patient harm.

As the field of minimally invasive dentistry continues to evolve, a holistic approach that combines technological innovation with a deep commitment to patient-centered care will be essential. Future trends will undoubtedly drive the development of new techniques and materials that align with the principles of minimally invasive dentistry, ensuring that the focus remains on preserving natural tooth structure, reducing patient discomfort, and enhancing overall treatment outcomes. The ongoing pursuit of excellence in dental care will be guided by the integration of cutting-edge technologies, advancements in biomaterials, and a commitment to personalized patient care, marking a new era in the practice of minimally invasive dentistry.

CHAPTER 15: IMPLEMENTING MINIMALLY INVASIVE TECHNIQUES IN CLINICAL PRACTICE

The integration of minimally invasive techniques into clinical practice represents a significant paradigm shift in dentistry. Embracing these techniques requires a comprehensive approach that extends beyond merely adopting new procedures; it necessitates a fundamental change in practice philosophy, staff training, and patient management. This chapter provides practical guidance on navigating this transition, ensuring that the adoption of minimally invasive practices is both effective and sustainable.

To begin with, transitioning from traditional to minimally invasive dentistry involves a thorough evaluation of current practice protocols and an understanding of how these new techniques align with the overall treatment goals. The first step in this process is to conduct an in-depth assessment of existing workflows and identify areas where minimally invasive techniques can be seamlessly integrated. This evaluation should include a review of current treatment methodologies, patient outcomes, and available resources.

Once areas for improvement are identified, the next critical step is to invest in staff training. Minimally invasive techniques often require new skills and a different approach to patient care. Training programs should be designed to cover not only the technical aspects of these procedures but also the underlying principles of minimally invasive dentistry. This includes educating staff on the benefits of preserving natural tooth structure, the use of advanced technologies, and the importance of patient-centered care. Workshops, hands-on training sessions, and continuing education courses can provide the necessary skills and knowledge to ensure that all team members are proficient in these new techniques.

In addition to technical training, it is essential to foster a cultural shift within the practice. Staff members should be encouraged to embrace the philosophy of minimally invasive dentistry and understand its impact on patient outcomes and overall practice success. This cultural shift can be supported through regular team meetings, case discussions, and the sharing of best practices. Open communication and collaboration among team members will help in addressing any challenges that arise during the implementation process and ensure that everyone is aligned with the new practice goals.

Adjusting workflows to accommodate minimally invasive techniques is another crucial aspect of the transition. This may involve re-evaluating and modifying existing protocols, investing in new equipment, and integrating digital technologies that support minimally invasive procedures. For example, the adoption of digital impressions and CAD/CAM systems may streamline restorative processes and enhance precision. Workflow adjustments should be carefully planned to minimize disruptions and ensure that all new procedures are integrated smoothly into the daily routine.

Patient communication is also a key factor in the successful implementation of minimally invasive techniques. Patients need to understand the benefits of these approaches, including reduced discomfort, shorter recovery times, and improved long-term outcomes. Effective communication strategies should be employed to educate patients about the advantages of minimally invasive treatments and address any concerns they may have. Informational materials, such as brochures and digital content, can be used to provide patients with clear and concise information about the procedures being offered.

Moreover, it is important to establish mechanisms for monitoring and evaluating the effectiveness of the newly implemented techniques. Regular assessment of patient outcomes, staff feedback, and procedural efficiency will help identify areas for improvement and ensure that the transition is meeting the desired objectives. Continuous quality improvement initiatives should be in place to address any issues that arise and to refine processes as needed.

The successful implementation of minimally invasive techniques also depends on the support and leadership of the dental practice's management. Leaders must be proactive in championing the adoption of these techniques, providing the necessary resources, and fostering an environment that supports innovation and excellence in patient care. Leadership should also be prepared to address any resistance to change and provide guidance and encouragement throughout the transition process.

Ultimately, the goal of integrating minimally invasive techniques into clinical practice is to enhance patient care while maintaining the highest standards of dental practice. By focusing on thorough training, workflow optimization, effective patient communication, and continuous evaluation, dental practices can achieve a smooth and successful transition to minimally invasive approaches. This transition not only benefits patients by offering more conservative and comfortable treatment options but also contributes to the overall success and reputation of the dental practice.

Successfully integrating minimally invasive techniques into a dental practice requires careful planning and execution. After laying the groundwork through staff training, workflow adjustments, and patient communication, the next step involves addressing the practicalities of incorporating these techniques into everyday clinical practice. This phase includes optimizing the use of technology, establishing protocols for new procedures, and ensuring that the entire team is on board with the transition.

One of the most significant aspects of adopting minimally invasive dentistry is the integration of advanced technologies. These technologies often require initial investment but can greatly enhance the efficiency and effectiveness of minimally invasive procedures. For example, digital impression systems and CAD/CAM technology streamline the process of creating restorations with high precision, reducing the need for traditional, more invasive methods. Practices must consider the compatibility of these technologies with their existing systems and workflows, ensuring that new equipment is seamlessly incorporated into daily operations.

Additionally, the implementation of laser systems and air abrasion technologies can further complement minimally invasive techniques. Lasers offer precise tissue removal with minimal discomfort, while air abrasion can effectively treat carious lesions with less removal of healthy tooth structure compared to traditional drills. Integrating these tools involves not only purchasing and maintaining the equipment but also ensuring that the clinical team is well-trained in their use. Practical training sessions and simulation exercises can help practitioners become adept at using these technologies, leading to improved patient outcomes and practice efficiency.

Protocols and procedures must also be updated to reflect the adoption of minimally invasive techniques. This involves creating or revising standard operating procedures that align with the new techniques being introduced. For instance, protocols for patient assessment, diagnosis, and treatment planning should be adapted to incorporate minimally invasive principles. These protocols must be clearly documented and communicated to all team members to ensure consistency and high-quality care across the practice. Regular reviews and updates to these protocols may be necessary as new technologies and techniques evolve.

An important part of the integration process is establishing clear lines of communication within the practice. Regular team meetings and briefings can facilitate the exchange of information about the progress of the implementation process, address any challenges encountered, and share insights and experiences. Encouraging feedback from staff members can provide valuable insights into the effectiveness of the new techniques and highlight areas for improvement. This collaborative approach helps in refining the implementation process and ensuring that all team members are engaged and supportive of the changes.

Patient management and communication also play a critical role in the successful integration of minimally invasive techniques. As these techniques often involve new approaches to treatment, it is essential to educate patients about the benefits and limitations of minimally invasive procedures. Informative consultations, visual aids, and detailed explanations can help patients understand how these techniques work and why they are advantageous compared to traditional methods. Addressing patient concerns and expectations proactively contributes to a positive experience and helps build trust in the new treatment approach.

Moreover, tracking and evaluating the outcomes of minimally invasive procedures is vital for continuous improvement. Implementing a system for monitoring treatment results, patient satisfaction, and procedural efficiency can provide data that informs future practice decisions. This may include collecting feedback from patients regarding their comfort and satisfaction with the new techniques, as well as assessing the clinical outcomes to ensure that the procedures are achieving the desired results. Regular analysis of this data allows for ongoing refinement of techniques and protocols, leading to better patient care and practice efficiency.

In addition to internal evaluation, practices should stay informed about advancements in minimally invasive dentistry and continuously seek opportunities for further education and training. This ongoing learning process ensures that the practice remains at the forefront of innovation and can adapt to new developments in the field. Attending professional conferences, participating in workshops, and subscribing to relevant dental journals are effective ways to keep abreast of emerging trends and technologies.

Finally, the successful integration of minimally invasive techniques into clinical practice is a dynamic process that requires commitment, flexibility, and a patient-centered approach. By embracing these principles and addressing the practical aspects of implementation, dental practices can enhance their ability to provide high-quality, conservative care. This approach not only benefits patients through improved outcomes and reduced discomfort but also positions the practice as a leader in modern, minimally invasive dental care.

A critical aspect of integrating minimally invasive techniques into clinical practice involves addressing the logistical and financial considerations that accompany the transition. Implementing these techniques often requires an initial investment in new equipment and technology, which can be a significant consideration for many practices. To manage these costs effectively, it is important to develop a comprehensive financial plan that considers both the short-term and long-term implications of the investment.

Practices may explore various financing options to support the acquisition of new technology, such as leasing equipment or applying for loans. Additionally, the financial benefits of minimally invasive techniques, including increased patient throughput and potentially reduced overhead costs associated with fewer post-operative complications, should be factored into the cost-benefit analysis. Evaluating these aspects helps in making informed decisions about the investment and ensures that the transition remains financially viable.

Once new technologies and techniques are in place, ongoing maintenance and support are essential to ensure their optimal performance. Establishing service contracts with equipment suppliers and technology providers can provide regular maintenance and prompt repairs, minimizing downtime and ensuring that the practice remains operational. Furthermore, it is beneficial to have a dedicated team member or practice administrator who oversees the maintenance and operation of these technologies, ensuring that any issues are addressed promptly.

The integration of minimally invasive techniques also involves modifying patient scheduling and workflow to accommodate the nuances of new procedures. For instance, procedures using digital impressions or CAD/CAM technology may require additional time for preparation and processing compared to traditional methods. Adjusting patient appointment schedules to account for these variations ensures that the practice operates efficiently while maintaining high standards of care.

Training and education extend beyond the initial phase of implementation. Continuous professional development is crucial as technologies and techniques evolve. Regular refresher courses and advanced training sessions can help staff members stay current with new developments and refine their skills. Incorporating this ongoing education into the practice's routine helps in maintaining high competency levels and ensures that the team is equipped to handle new challenges as they arise.

Another important consideration is the adaptation of patient management strategies to align with the principles of minimally invasive dentistry. Engaging patients in their own care by educating them about the benefits and procedures associated with minimally invasive techniques fosters a collaborative approach. Patients who understand the advantages of these techniques, such as reduced discomfort and faster recovery times, are more likely to engage positively with the treatment process and adhere to recommended care plans.

Communication with patients should be clear, concise, and empathetic. Providing detailed explanations about the procedures, what they entail, and how they differ from traditional methods helps in setting realistic expectations. Utilizing visual aids and digital simulations can further enhance patient understanding and comfort. Ensuring that patients are well-informed and comfortable with their treatment choices contributes to higher satisfaction rates and improved clinical outcomes.

Additionally, integrating patient feedback into the practice's approach is valuable for continuous improvement. Regularly soliciting feedback through surveys or direct conversations can provide insights into patient experiences with minimally invasive procedures. Analyzing this feedback allows practices to identify areas for improvement and make necessary adjustments to enhance the overall patient experience.

The broader implications of adopting minimally invasive techniques also involve contributing to the advancement of the field. Practices that successfully implement these techniques can serve as models for other practitioners and contribute to the dissemination of knowledge and best practices within the dental community. Participating in professional forums, publishing case studies, and engaging in collaborative research initiatives are ways to share experiences and advance the practice of minimally invasive dentistry.

In conclusion, the successful implementation of minimally invasive techniques in a clinical setting requires a multifaceted approach that encompasses financial planning, staff training, workflow adjustments, patient communication, and ongoing professional development. By addressing these areas comprehensively, dental practices can achieve a smooth transition to minimally invasive methods, ultimately enhancing patient care and practice efficiency. The commitment to continuous improvement and adaptation ensures that the practice remains at the forefront of modern dentistry, providing high-quality, conservative care that meets the evolving needs of patients.

CHAPTER 16: CLINICAL CASE STUDIES IN MINIMALLY INVASIVE DENTISTRY

In this chapter, a series of clinical case studies are presented to provide a detailed examination of minimally invasive techniques applied across various dental scenarios. These case studies offer a practical perspective on the challenges and solutions associated with adopting minimally invasive approaches, showcasing their impact on patient care and clinical outcomes.

The first case study focuses on a patient with early-stage carious lesions on multiple teeth. Traditional approaches might have involved extensive tooth preparation and restoration, but the minimally invasive strategy emphasized the use of microdentistry and resin infiltration. The patient presented with incipient carious lesions primarily in the interproximal areas of the anterior teeth. Conventional treatment would likely involve substantial enamel removal, risking the vitality of the tooth and leading to more significant restorations. However, employing a minimally invasive approach, the treatment team utilized resin infiltration to arrest carious progression without significant tooth reduction.

The initial step in this case was the application of a mild acid etchant to the affected areas to increase the porosity of the carious lesions. This process allowed the resin infiltrant to penetrate the carious dentin more effectively. The application was followed by curing with a light-activated polymerization device, ensuring that the resin set properly and formed a robust barrier against further carious activity. The outcome was successful, with the lesions halting in progression and the patient reporting no discomfort or need for more invasive procedures. This case underscores how minimally invasive techniques can preserve tooth structure and provide an effective treatment alternative for early carious lesions.

In another case study, a patient with significant dental erosion due to acidic dietary habits was treated using a combination of remineralization strategies and conservative restorative techniques. The erosion had led to considerable loss of enamel and dentin, particularly on the buccal surfaces of the molars. Traditional restorative approaches might have required extensive reconstruction with crowns or large restorations. Instead, the minimally invasive strategy focused on preventive and conservative measures.

The treatment plan included a comprehensive assessment of the patient's dietary habits and oral hygiene practices. Recommendations were made to modify dietary intake, reduce acid exposure, and enhance fluoride use to aid in enamel remineralization. In conjunction, the patient received conservative composite restorations to address the areas of significant loss and protect the underlying tooth structure. The restoration process was carefully managed to ensure minimal reduction of existing tooth structure, using bonded resin composites to restore function and aesthetics. This approach not only provided immediate relief and protection but also addressed the underlying issue of erosion through preventive measures.

Another compelling case involved a patient presenting with severe attrition due to bruxism. The wear patterns were extensive, affecting multiple teeth and leading to functional and esthetic concerns. Traditionally, such cases would often necessitate extensive restorations or even occlusal adjustments. However, the minimally invasive approach aimed to address the issue with less invasive methods.

For this patient, a combination of occlusal splints and conservative restorations was employed. The occlusal splints were designed to mitigate the effects of bruxism and protect the teeth from further attrition. Conservative composite buildups were utilized to restore the lost tooth structure, with careful attention to occlusal adjustments to avoid exacerbating the bruxism. Additionally, patient education on stress management and bruxism prevention strategies was provided to address the underlying cause. The outcome was positive, with restored function and aesthetics, reduced wear progression, and improved patient satisfaction.

In a final case study, the focus was on a patient with periodontal tissue loss and subsequent exposure of root surfaces, which could complicate restorative efforts. Traditional treatments might have involved extensive surgical interventions or the placement of large restorations. The minimally invasive approach utilized regenerative techniques and conservative restoration methods to manage the tissue loss effectively.

The treatment plan involved the use of advanced regenerative materials, including platelet-rich fibrin (PRF) and bioactive glass, to promote tissue healing and regeneration. The application of these materials was carefully planned to stimulate the growth of new periodontal tissue and enhance the structural support of the teeth. Conservative composite restorations were then applied to cover the exposed root surfaces and protect against further damage. This case highlighted the potential of minimally invasive techniques to achieve functional and esthetic outcomes while preserving as much natural tooth structure and supporting tissues as possible.

These clinical case studies collectively illustrate the diverse applications and benefits of minimally invasive techniques in dentistry. By focusing on preservation, conservation, and conservative treatment approaches, these cases demonstrate how minimally invasive methods can address various dental conditions effectively. Each case offers valuable insights into the practical aspects of implementing these techniques, providing a foundation for practitioners to consider when adopting minimally invasive strategies in their own practices.

In another detailed case study, a patient presented with multiple carious lesions and severe hypersensitivity in several premolars. The traditional approach might have involved extensive tooth preparation and placement of large restorations. However, applying minimally invasive techniques focused on preserving as much of the natural tooth structure as possible while addressing the sensitivity.

Initial diagnostic procedures included comprehensive clinical examination and diagnostic imaging to assess the extent of carious lesions and underlying dentin sensitivity. To address the hypersensitivity, a treatment strategy was devised that integrated both restorative and desensitizing measures. The minimally invasive approach included the application of fluoride varnishes and desensitizing agents to reduce sensitivity before initiating restorative procedures.

For the carious lesions, the approach involved selective carious removal using microdentistry techniques. This technique allows for the precise removal of carious tissue while preserving as much healthy dentin as possible. The cavities were then treated with resin-based composite materials to restore tooth structure and function. The use of adhesive bonding agents ensured a strong bond between the tooth and restorative material, minimizing the risk of future sensitivity and promoting long-term success. This case exemplifies how minimally invasive techniques can manage complex conditions effectively while prioritizing tooth preservation and patient comfort.

A different scenario involved a patient with significant enamel erosion attributed to chronic acid reflux. The erosion had led to significant loss of tooth structure, affecting both the aesthetics and function of the teeth. The traditional approach might have required extensive crowns or veneers. Instead, the minimally invasive strategy focused on conservative restorative techniques and preventive measures.

The treatment plan began with addressing the underlying cause of the enamel erosion through medical consultation and lifestyle modifications to manage acid reflux. In conjunction with these measures, the patient received conservative restorations with resin-based composites. These restorations were designed to rebuild lost enamel while maintaining a natural appearance. The use of fluoride treatments and remineralization agents was also recommended to enhance the recovery of remaining enamel and prevent further erosion. This case highlights the effectiveness of minimally invasive techniques in managing extensive enamel loss by combining conservative restorations with preventive care.

Another case study explored the application of minimally invasive techniques in managing early-stage periodontal disease. The patient presented with gingival inflammation and initial periodontal pocket formation. Traditionally, such conditions might have warranted more invasive surgical interventions. However, a minimally invasive approach was utilized to address the periodontal issues through non-surgical methods.

The treatment included a thorough scaling and root planing procedure, using ultrasonic and hand instruments to meticulously remove plaque and calculus without causing excessive tissue trauma. Additionally, antimicrobial agents were used to manage infection and promote healing. The patient was also provided with detailed oral hygiene instructions and a customized home care regimen to support the non-surgical management of periodontal disease. Regular follow-up visits were scheduled to monitor progress and adjust treatment as necessary. This case underscores the value of minimally invasive periodontal techniques in effectively managing early-stage disease while minimizing patient discomfort and promoting long-term oral health.

In a final case, a patient with severe bruxism and resultant tooth wear presented for treatment. The bruxism had caused significant attrition of the occlusal surfaces of the posterior teeth. Traditional approaches might have involved the use of extensive crowns or occlusal adjustments. However, the minimally invasive approach focused on conservative management strategies and preventive care.

The treatment plan included the fabrication of a custom occlusal splint to protect the teeth from further wear and manage bruxism. Conservative composite restorations were used to restore the occlusal surfaces of the worn teeth, with careful attention given to occlusal adjustments to ensure proper function and alignment. Additionally, the patient received counseling on stress management techniques to address the underlying causes of bruxism. The outcome was favorable, with restored tooth function and aesthetics and reduced progression of tooth wear. This case highlights the potential of minimally invasive techniques to manage complex dental issues by combining conservative restorative methods with preventive and supportive care.

These case studies collectively demonstrate the practical application and benefits of minimally invasive techniques in diverse clinical scenarios. They illustrate how these approaches can be effectively employed to manage a range of dental conditions while prioritizing tooth preservation, patient comfort, and long-term success. Each case provides valuable insights into the real-world application of minimally invasive dentistry, offering guidance for clinicians seeking to integrate these techniques into their practice.

In a final case study, we examine the treatment of a patient presenting with a large carious lesion in a molar that had been previously filled with a traditional amalgam restoration. The lesion extended close to the pulp, presenting a significant challenge in preserving tooth vitality while managing the extensive decay. The traditional approach might have involved root canal therapy followed by a large crown, potentially sacrificing significant tooth structure.

The minimally invasive strategy, however, focused on preserving as much of the natural tooth as possible while addressing the carious lesion effectively. Initial steps included a detailed diagnostic assessment through radiographic imaging to evaluate the extent of decay and the proximity to the pulp. The carious tissue was carefully removed using precision dental instruments to avoid unnecessary damage to the surrounding healthy dentin.

Instead of a conventional root canal procedure, a more conservative approach was employed. The tooth was treated with a selective removal of decayed tissue followed by pulp capping, a technique designed to protect the pulp and stimulate repair of the dentin. A calcium hydroxide liner was applied to provide a protective barrier and encourage secondary dentin formation. The cavity was then restored with a resin-based composite material, carefully layered to match the natural anatomy of the tooth and ensure a strong bond with the remaining structure. This approach successfully preserved the majority of the tooth structure, maintained vitality, and provided a durable restoration. This case highlights how minimally invasive techniques can effectively manage complex carious lesions while minimizing invasive procedures and preserving tooth integrity.

Another illustrative case involved a patient with severe dental fluorosis, presenting with intrinsic staining and enamel hypoplasia. The aesthetic impact of fluorosis was significant, affecting the patient's smile and overall confidence. Traditional treatment options might have included extensive porcelain veneers or crowns, which could be invasive and costly.

The minimally invasive approach for this case involved the use of microabrasion and bleaching techniques to improve the appearance of the fluorosed teeth. Microabrasion was employed to remove a thin layer of stained enamel, followed by a professional whitening procedure to address the intrinsic discoloration. This conservative approach effectively improved the aesthetic appearance of the teeth without extensive preparation or the need for more invasive restorative options. For the final touch, a minimal-layered composite veneer was used to enhance the aesthetics further while preserving the natural tooth structure. This case underscores the efficacy of minimally invasive techniques in managing aesthetic concerns with minimal alteration to the natural tooth structure.

In another case, a patient with a history of dental trauma presented with a fractured anterior tooth. The traditional approach might have involved the placement of a full-coverage crown to restore the tooth's function and appearance. However, the minimally invasive approach focused on a more conservative method.

The treatment involved the use of direct resin bonding to repair the fractured tooth. The fractured area was meticulously cleaned and prepared, and a composite resin was applied to restore the tooth's shape and function. The resin was carefully layered and sculpted to match the natural contours and shade of the tooth, resulting in a restoration that was both aesthetically pleasing and functionally effective. This method not only preserved the natural tooth structure but also avoided the need for more invasive crown preparation. The patient's satisfaction with the outcome and the preservation of tooth structure were significant benefits of this minimally invasive approach.

In yet another scenario, a patient presented with multiple abraded teeth due to excessive brushing with a hard-bristled toothbrush. The abraded areas were sensitive and aesthetically unpleasing. Traditionally, such cases might have been addressed with extensive restorative treatments, including crowns or large composite restorations.

The minimally invasive approach involved the use of a combination of resin-based fillings and preventive measures. The abraded areas were restored with a flowable composite material, which was chosen for its ability to adapt well to the tooth surface and provide a seamless restoration. Additionally, the patient was advised on proper brushing techniques and the use of a softer toothbrush to prevent further abrasion. This case demonstrates how a minimally invasive approach can effectively manage sensitivity and aesthetic issues while promoting better oral hygiene practices to prevent recurrence.

These case studies collectively illustrate the practical application and benefits of minimally invasive techniques in diverse clinical scenarios. They provide valuable insights into how these approaches can be effectively utilized to manage a range of dental conditions while prioritizing tooth preservation and patient comfort. Each case highlights the importance of tailoring treatment strategies to the specific needs of the patient, demonstrating how minimally invasive techniques can achieve excellent outcomes with a conservative approach.

CHAPTER 17: MINIMALLY INVASIVE TECHNIQUES FOR AESTHETIC DENTISTRY

Aesthetic dentistry continually evolves with the goal of enhancing smile appearance while minimizing the impact on natural tooth structure. Minimally invasive techniques play a pivotal role in this field, offering advanced solutions for improving dental aesthetics with greater preservation of tooth integrity. This chapter delves into several such techniques, highlighting their application in various aesthetic procedures, including tooth whitening, veneer placements, and cosmetic bonding.

Tooth whitening, or bleaching, is one of the most common minimally invasive aesthetic procedures. It is a conservative approach that can significantly enhance the appearance of teeth without the need for extensive intervention. The process involves the application of bleaching agents, typically containing hydrogen peroxide or carbamide peroxide, to the tooth surface. These agents work by penetrating the enamel and breaking down the stains and discolorations within the tooth structure. Professional whitening treatments can be performed in-office or at home, with custom-made trays provided for at-home use. In-office treatments, often utilizing higher concentrations of bleaching agents, can produce immediate results and are particularly effective for patients with significant staining.

Tooth whitening is generally well-tolerated and is considered a minimally invasive procedure as it does not require the removal of tooth structure. However, it is crucial to evaluate the patient's oral health before proceeding, as whitening may not be suitable for individuals with certain conditions such as active periodontal disease or extensive restorations. Additionally, sensitivity during and after the whitening process is a common side effect, but it is typically transient and manageable with appropriate desensitizing treatments.

Another minimally invasive approach in aesthetic dentistry is the use of veneers. Veneers are thin, custom-made shells that cover the front surface of teeth to improve their appearance. They are typically crafted from porcelain or composite resin and are bonded to the tooth surface. The application of veneers is less invasive compared to traditional crowns, as it requires only minimal reduction of tooth structure, primarily to create space for the veneer and to ensure a proper fit.

Porcelain veneers are highly valued for their durability and ability to mimic the natural translucency of tooth enamel. They are an excellent option for correcting a variety of aesthetic issues, including discoloration, chipping, and gaps between teeth. The process involves an initial consultation, where the desired outcome is discussed, followed by tooth preparation and impression taking. The impressions are sent to a dental laboratory, where the veneers are fabricated. Once ready, the veneers are bonded to the teeth with a strong adhesive, resulting in a natural-looking and aesthetically pleasing enhancement.

Composite resin veneers, on the other hand, offer a more cost-effective and less invasive alternative. These veneers are applied directly to the tooth surface and sculpted to achieve the desired shape and color. The process can often be completed in a single visit, making it a convenient option for patients seeking quick results. Composite veneers are particularly useful for minor cosmetic corrections and can be easily adjusted or replaced if necessary.

Cosmetic bonding is another minimally invasive technique that involves the application of tooth-colored resin to repair and enhance the appearance of teeth. The resin is applied to the tooth surface, shaped, and then hardened using a special light. This technique is ideal for addressing minor imperfections such as chips, gaps, or irregularities in tooth shape. Cosmetic bonding is often chosen for its simplicity and versatility, allowing for immediate results with minimal impact on the natural tooth structure.

The application of cosmetic bonding is straightforward and generally requires no or minimal tooth preparation. The resin is carefully matched to the tooth color to ensure a seamless blend with the surrounding teeth. The process is highly conservative, making it suitable for patients who wish to address aesthetic concerns without significant alteration to their natural teeth. Additionally, cosmetic bonding can be used in combination with other treatments, such as tooth whitening or veneers, to achieve a comprehensive aesthetic improvement.

Minimally invasive techniques in aesthetic dentistry not only prioritize the preservation of tooth structure but also emphasize patient comfort and satisfaction. Advances in materials and technology have enhanced the efficacy and precision of these treatments, allowing for more predictable and durable outcomes. The integration of these techniques into clinical practice represents a significant advancement in aesthetic dentistry, offering patients the opportunity to achieve their desired smile while maintaining the integrity of their natural teeth.

In summary, minimally invasive techniques for aesthetic dentistry provide a range of options for enhancing smile aesthetics with minimal impact on tooth structure. Tooth whitening, veneers, and cosmetic bonding are effective methods for improving dental appearance, each offering distinct advantages and tailored solutions for various aesthetic concerns. As the field of aesthetic dentistry continues to evolve, the focus on minimally invasive approaches ensures that patients can achieve optimal results while preserving their natural dental health.

In addition to tooth whitening, veneer placements, and cosmetic bonding, minimally invasive techniques in aesthetic dentistry also encompass a range of other approaches designed to enhance the appearance of the smile while preserving natural tooth structure. One such technique is the use of microabrasion, which is particularly effective for treating superficial dental discoloration and enamel imperfections.

Microabrasion involves the application of a fine abrasive agent, often combined with an acidic solution, to the surface of the tooth. This method removes a thin layer of the outer enamel, thereby eliminating surface stains and improving the tooth's overall appearance. It is especially beneficial for patients with intrinsic stains or enamel defects that cannot be addressed with conventional whitening methods. The procedure is minimally invasive as it targets only the outermost layer of the tooth without affecting the underlying dentin.

Another minimally invasive approach gaining popularity is the use of digital smile design (DSD) technology. DSD allows for a comprehensive digital assessment and planning of aesthetic treatments. By using digital imaging and computer-aided design software, clinicians can create highly accurate visual simulations of potential outcomes before initiating any treatment. This technology enables precise planning and customization of aesthetic procedures such as veneers and crowns, ensuring that the final result aligns closely with the patient's expectations. Moreover, DSD facilitates communication between the clinician and the patient, providing a clear visual representation of the anticipated changes and allowing for better-informed decisions.

The application of laser technology in aesthetic dentistry also represents a significant advancement in minimally invasive techniques. Lasers can be used for a variety of purposes, including tooth whitening, gum contouring, and treatment of oral soft tissue lesions. The precision and control offered by lasers minimize damage to surrounding tissues and reduce postoperative discomfort. For instance, in gum contouring procedures, lasers can reshape the gum line with minimal bleeding and faster healing compared to traditional surgical methods. Similarly, lasers used in tooth whitening enhance the efficacy of bleaching agents and expedite the whitening process.

Furthermore, the development of advanced adhesive technologies has revolutionized minimally invasive aesthetic procedures. Modern dental adhesives provide strong bonding capabilities with minimal preparation, allowing for the application of veneers and bonding materials with reduced removal of tooth structure. These adhesives enhance the longevity and durability of aesthetic restorations while preserving the natural tooth. Their use is particularly important in techniques such as direct composite restorations, where the adhesive plays a crucial role in ensuring a seamless integration of the composite material with the tooth structure.

Innovative materials such as nano-composites have also contributed to the advancement of minimally invasive aesthetic dentistry. Nano-composites are resin-based materials that incorporate nanoparticles to improve their mechanical properties and esthetic qualities. These materials offer superior strength, wear resistance, and color stability compared to traditional composites. They are ideal for use in cosmetic bonding and veneer applications, providing a natural appearance and excellent performance while minimizing the need for extensive tooth preparation.

In the realm of smile design, digital photography and imaging play a critical role in planning and executing aesthetic procedures. High-resolution digital photographs allow for detailed analysis of the smile and help in assessing factors such as tooth proportion, alignment, and symmetry. These images can be used to create diagnostic mock-ups, which are valuable for visualizing potential outcomes and making necessary adjustments before proceeding with treatment. Digital imaging also aids in monitoring the progress of ongoing treatments and ensuring that the results meet the desired aesthetic goals.

The integration of minimally invasive techniques in aesthetic dentistry not only enhances the visual appeal of the smile but also aligns with the broader principles of conservative dental care. By focusing on preserving natural tooth structure and employing less invasive methods, these techniques contribute to improved patient comfort and satisfaction. The emphasis on conservative approaches allows for the achievement of optimal esthetic outcomes while minimizing the risk of adverse effects and the need for more invasive procedures in the future.

In conclusion, the field of minimally invasive aesthetic dentistry encompasses a diverse array of techniques and technologies aimed at enhancing smile aesthetics while preserving natural tooth structure. Methods such as tooth whitening, veneer placements, cosmetic bonding, microabrasion, digital smile design, laser treatments, advanced adhesives, and nano-composites represent significant advancements in achieving aesthetic improvements with minimal intervention. As the field continues to evolve, these techniques offer patients the opportunity to achieve their desired smile outcomes while maintaining the health and integrity of their natural teeth.

In exploring minimally invasive techniques for aesthetic dentistry, it is important to understand how these approaches align with contemporary goals of preserving tooth structure while achieving high-quality esthetic results. A key factor in this alignment is the development and use of advanced diagnostic tools that facilitate precise treatment planning and execution.

Digital scanning technologies have transformed the way aesthetic treatments are planned and executed. Intraoral scanners, for instance, provide highly accurate digital impressions that eliminate the discomfort and inaccuracies associated with traditional impression materials. These digital impressions allow for the creation of precise models used in the fabrication of restorations such as veneers and crowns. By utilizing digital models, clinicians can achieve better-fitting restorations with minimal adjustments, thereby preserving more of the natural tooth structure and enhancing patient comfort.

The advent of virtual smile design is another significant advancement in aesthetic dentistry. Virtual smile design software enables clinicians to visualize and plan the final esthetic outcome before initiating any physical alterations to the teeth. Through the use of digital photographs and 3D imaging, this technology allows for detailed simulation of proposed changes, helping both the dentist and the patient to make informed decisions. The ability to preview potential outcomes and make adjustments in the digital realm helps ensure that the final result meets the patient's expectations and adheres to aesthetic standards.

In addition to digital tools, advancements in bonding materials have played a crucial role in minimizing the invasiveness of aesthetic procedures. Modern bonding agents provide strong adhesion with minimal preparation, allowing for the application of esthetic materials like composite resins and veneers with minimal alteration to the tooth structure. The development of self-etching adhesives and improved resin formulations has further enhanced the effectiveness of bonding, resulting in more durable and aesthetically pleasing restorations.

The use of tooth-colored materials, such as advanced composites and ceramics, has also contributed to the minimally invasive approach in aesthetic dentistry. These materials are designed to closely match the natural color and translucency of tooth enamel, resulting in restorations that blend seamlessly with the surrounding teeth. Innovations in material science have led to the development of highly aesthetic and functional materials that can be applied with minimal tooth preparation.

For patients seeking smile enhancement, the role of cosmetic bonding has become increasingly prominent. Cosmetic bonding involves the application of tooth-colored resins to correct imperfections such as chips, gaps, and minor misalignments. This technique is less invasive compared to traditional restorative methods, as it requires minimal tooth alteration and can often be completed in a single visit. The versatility of bonding materials allows for customized solutions that address specific esthetic concerns while preserving the natural tooth structure.

Another area where minimally invasive techniques have made significant strides is in the treatment of tooth discoloration. Professional tooth whitening remains one of the most sought-after cosmetic procedures, and recent advancements have improved its effectiveness and safety. Modern whitening systems utilize advanced formulations and delivery methods that achieve superior results with reduced sensitivity. These systems often include custom-fitted trays or in-office treatments that provide controlled application of whitening agents, ensuring even and predictable outcomes.

In addition to these techniques, preventive measures play a crucial role in maintaining aesthetic results and overall oral health. Regular dental check-ups, professional cleanings, and adherence to good oral hygiene practices are essential in preventing issues that may compromise the results of aesthetic treatments. Preventive care helps to address potential problems early, minimizing the need for more invasive interventions and ensuring that esthetic enhancements are maintained over time.

In summary, the application of minimally invasive techniques in aesthetic dentistry reflects a commitment to preserving natural tooth structure while achieving optimal esthetic outcomes. Through advancements in digital imaging, virtual smile design, bonding materials, and tooth-colored restorations, clinicians can provide patients with high-quality cosmetic enhancements that align with contemporary standards of care. These techniques not only enhance the appearance of the smile but also contribute to overall patient satisfaction by offering less invasive, more comfortable, and more predictable solutions for achieving a beautiful and healthy smile.

CHAPTER 18: THE ROLE OF LASER TECHNOLOGY IN MINIMALLY INVASIVE DENTISTRY

Laser technology has increasingly become a significant component in the practice of minimally invasive dentistry, offering innovative solutions that align with the principles of preserving tooth structure and enhancing patient comfort. This chapter provides an in-depth exploration of how lasers are applied in dental procedures, highlighting their benefits in soft tissue management, caries removal, and periodontal treatments. The emphasis is on how laser technology contributes to precision, efficiency, and patient satisfaction, revolutionizing traditional approaches to dental care.

Lasers operate on the principle of stimulating atoms or molecules to emit light at a specific wavelength. This light is concentrated into a beam that can be precisely directed to perform various functions in dentistry. The effectiveness of a laser depends on its wavelength, which determines its interaction with different types of tissue. For instance, the Er:YAG laser, with its ability to effectively remove hard tissues, is commonly used for cavity preparation and enamel removal.

Conversely, the diode laser, known for its efficiency with soft tissues, is frequently employed in procedures such as gingival contouring and biopsy.

In the realm of soft tissue management, lasers offer substantial advantages over traditional surgical methods. One of the key benefits is their precision. Lasers provide a high degree of control over the depth and extent of tissue removal, allowing for more conservative interventions. This precision minimizes collateral damage to surrounding healthy tissues, reducing post-operative discomfort and promoting faster healing. For example, in periodontal therapy, lasers can selectively target diseased tissue and bacteria while sparing the healthy gum tissue. This targeted approach not only enhances the efficacy of the treatment but also contributes to a more comfortable recovery for the patient.

The use of lasers in caries removal represents another significant advancement in minimally invasive dentistry. Traditional methods of caries removal, such as drilling, often involve the removal of healthy tooth structure along with the decayed portion. In contrast, lasers can selectively target and remove carious dentin with minimal impact on the surrounding healthy tooth structure. This selectivity allows for more conservative preparation of cavities, preserving as much of the natural tooth as possible. Additionally, laser treatments can often be performed without the need for anesthesia, further enhancing patient comfort and reducing the need for invasive procedures.

The application of laser technology extends to various aspects of periodontal treatment. Lasers are used in scaling and root planing to remove calculus and smooth the root surfaces, facilitating the healing of the periodontal tissues. The antimicrobial properties of lasers also help in reducing bacterial load, which is crucial for managing periodontal disease. Moreover, lasers can be utilized in the treatment of gingival hyperplasia, a condition characterized by overgrowth of gum tissue. By precisely targeting and excising the excess tissue, lasers offer a minimally invasive solution that minimizes discomfort and promotes quicker healing compared to traditional surgical methods.

Beyond their clinical applications, lasers contribute to the overall patient experience in minimally invasive dentistry. The use of lasers often results in less bleeding, reduced swelling, and minimal post-operative pain. This improved patient comfort can lead to higher satisfaction and better compliance with follow-up care. The non-contact nature of laser procedures also reduces the risk of cross-contamination, enhancing the safety of dental treatments. Additionally, the ability to perform procedures with minimal noise and vibration further alleviates patient anxiety, creating a more pleasant and less stressful dental experience.

As with any technology, the effective integration of lasers into dental practice requires a thorough understanding of their capabilities and limitations. Dentists must be trained in the specific applications of laser technology to ensure its safe and effective use. This training encompasses not only the technical aspects of operating lasers but also the clinical indications for their use and the interpretation of treatment outcomes. Continuing education and hands-on experience are essential for staying current with advancements in laser technology and maximizing its benefits in clinical practice.

In summary, laser technology represents a significant advancement in minimally invasive dentistry, offering numerous benefits that align with the principles of preserving tooth structure and enhancing patient comfort. Through their precise application in soft tissue management, caries removal, and periodontal treatments, lasers contribute to more conservative, effective, and comfortable dental care. The integration of lasers into dental practice requires careful consideration and training, but the potential benefits for both clinicians and patients make them a valuable tool in the pursuit of optimal dental health.

The application of laser technology in minimally invasive dentistry extends beyond its immediate clinical benefits to encompass aspects of procedural efficiency and patient experience. The ability of lasers to target specific tissues with precision translates into less invasive procedures and improved outcomes. By examining these advanced technologies, one can appreciate how lasers are transforming traditional dental practices, enhancing both procedural efficacy and patient comfort.

In the realm of caries management, lasers offer a marked improvement over conventional methods. Traditional drills used in restorative dentistry can be invasive, often resulting in the removal of healthy tooth structure along with decayed material. In contrast, lasers operate with selective absorption, meaning they can precisely target and vaporize carious tissue without unnecessarily compromising the surrounding healthy dentin. This selectivity not only aids in preserving natural tooth structure but also reduces the overall discomfort experienced by patients during and after the procedure. Additionally, the reduced need for anesthesia in many laser-assisted procedures contributes to a more comfortable patient experience and shorter recovery times.

The process of using lasers for caries removal begins with the selection of the appropriate laser wavelength. Different wavelengths are absorbed by different tissues, making it crucial to choose a laser that is specifically suited for the type of tissue being treated. For instance, the Er:YAG laser, which emits light at a wavelength of 2.94 micrometers, is particularly effective for hard tissue procedures such as cavity preparation. This laser's energy is absorbed by water and hydroxyapatite in the tooth structure, making it effective for caries removal while preserving surrounding healthy tissue. Furthermore, the precision of the laser beam allows for more controlled removal of carious dentin, which is essential for achieving optimal restoration outcomes.

When it comes to soft tissue management, lasers provide a versatile tool for a variety of procedures, from gingival contouring to frenectomy. The diode laser, for example, operates at a wavelength that is highly absorbed by hemoglobin and melanin, making it ideal for cutting and coagulating soft tissues with minimal bleeding. This characteristic is particularly beneficial for procedures involving the removal of excess gum tissue or reshaping the gingiva for aesthetic or functional purposes. The reduced bleeding and swelling associated with laser treatment contribute to a more comfortable recovery and a lower risk of post-operative complications.

Moreover, the application of lasers in periodontal therapy represents a significant advancement in managing periodontal disease. Lasers can be used to perform scaling and root planing, where the laser energy assists in removing calculus and smoothing root surfaces. The antimicrobial effects of lasers help in reducing the bacterial load within the periodontal pockets, which is crucial for the effective management of periodontal infections. By targeting diseased tissue and bacteria while preserving healthy tissue, lasers offer a minimally invasive alternative to traditional mechanical debridement methods. This selective removal of diseased tissue, coupled with the laser's ability to promote tissue regeneration, enhances the overall efficacy of periodontal treatment.

The benefits of laser technology extend to patient comfort and procedural efficiency as well. Laser procedures are often less noisy and cause less vibration compared to traditional dental drills, reducing patient anxiety and discomfort. The non-contact nature of lasers also minimizes the need for physical contact with the tooth or soft tissue, further enhancing patient comfort. Additionally, the precision of laser technology reduces the risk of damage to adjacent tissues, contributing to more predictable and favorable treatment outcomes.

Incorporating laser technology into clinical practice requires not only an understanding of the principles behind laser operation but also proficiency in its practical applications. Dentists must undergo specialized training to effectively utilize lasers for various procedures, ensuring that they are aware of the specific parameters and techniques required for optimal results. This training includes understanding the different types of lasers, their wavelengths, and their interactions with various tissues, as well as mastering the proper techniques for energy delivery and tissue manipulation.

The integration of lasers into a dental practice also involves considerations related to equipment and safety. Dentists must ensure that their practice is equipped with the appropriate laser devices and that all staff are trained in their use. Safety protocols must be established to protect both patients and dental professionals from potential hazards associated with laser use, such as eye injury from laser beams or exposure to laser-generated plumes. Proper protective eyewear and ventilation systems are essential components of a safe laser treatment environment.

In summary, laser technology has become a pivotal tool in minimally invasive dentistry, offering substantial advantages in terms of precision, patient comfort, and procedural efficiency. The ability to perform targeted interventions with minimal impact on surrounding tissues enhances the effectiveness of dental treatments while promoting a more comfortable patient experience. As dental practices continue to evolve, the role of lasers in minimally invasive techniques is likely to expand, further advancing the field and improving patient care.

As dental technology continues to advance, the integration of lasers into clinical practice represents a profound shift towards more precise, patient-friendly treatments. The impact of laser technology in minimally invasive dentistry extends beyond its immediate procedural benefits to include enhanced diagnostic capabilities and improvements in post-treatment care.

One notable application of laser technology is its role in the early detection and management of dental caries. Traditional methods of caries detection often rely on visual and tactile assessments, which can miss early-stage lesions. However, lasers equipped with specific wavelengths, such as the Diode or Nd:YAG lasers, can be used in conjunction with diagnostic systems to detect carious lesions at very early stages. These lasers can penetrate the tooth structure and detect changes in fluorescence associated with demineralization before they are visible or detectable with conventional methods. This capability allows for earlier intervention, potentially preventing the progression of carious lesions and minimizing the need for more invasive treatments.

In addition to detection, lasers have shown promise in the treatment of hypersensitivity, a common issue that can arise following dental procedures or due to environmental factors. Laser therapy for hypersensitivity involves the application of low-intensity lasers to the affected area, where the laser energy is absorbed by the dentinal tubules. This absorption helps to occlude the tubules and reduce the transmission of stimuli, providing relief from the discomfort associated with tooth sensitivity. This approach is particularly advantageous as it offers a non-invasive alternative to more traditional treatments, such as the application of desensitizing agents or restorations.

Furthermore, laser technology has been explored for its potential benefits in cosmetic dental procedures. For instance, the use of lasers for teeth whitening has gained popularity due to their ability to accelerate the whitening process and enhance results. The laser's light energy activates whitening agents more efficiently, leading to faster and more noticeable improvements in tooth color. This application aligns with the minimally invasive ethos by avoiding the need for aggressive mechanical whitening methods that can cause enamel abrasion or sensitivity.

In soft tissue procedures, lasers have revolutionized approaches to aesthetic enhancements and functional corrections. Techniques such as laser-assisted gingival contouring or crown lengthening are performed with remarkable precision, allowing for meticulous reshaping of the gingiva with minimal discomfort and rapid healing. By targeting specific tissue types and utilizing the laser's coagulation properties, practitioners can achieve desired aesthetic outcomes while preserving surrounding tissues and minimizing postoperative complications.

The role of lasers in periodontal therapy also highlights their efficacy in managing chronic periodontal diseases. The use of lasers in scaling and root planing procedures provides a thorough removal of bacterial deposits and calculus with enhanced precision. Lasers can selectively target diseased tissue within the periodontal pockets while promoting the regeneration of healthy tissue. This approach contributes to a more effective and less invasive treatment, improving patient outcomes and reducing the need for more extensive surgical interventions.

As dental practices adopt laser technology, considerations related to clinical implementation and patient safety must be addressed. Effective integration requires a comprehensive understanding of the different types of lasers available, their specific applications, and the proper techniques for their use. Additionally, ongoing training and adherence to safety protocols are essential for ensuring that laser treatments are conducted effectively and safely.

Practitioners must also stay abreast of emerging research and technological advancements in the field of laser dentistry. Continuous professional development ensures that dental professionals remain informed about the latest innovations and best practices, allowing them to provide the highest standard of care to their patients.

In summary, laser technology plays a transformative role in minimally invasive dentistry, offering significant advancements in precision, patient comfort, and procedural outcomes. The ability to perform targeted interventions with minimal impact on surrounding tissues enhances the effectiveness of various dental treatments while contributing to a more positive patient experience. As the field of laser dentistry continues to evolve, its integration into clinical practice will likely expand, further advancing the potential for minimally invasive techniques and improving patient care.

CHAPTER 19: ADDRESSING SENSITIVITY IN MINIMALLY INVASIVE TREATMENTS

Tooth sensitivity is a common concern in minimally invasive dentistry, where the emphasis on conserving tooth structure and avoiding extensive treatments can sometimes lead to discomfort or heightened sensitivity in patients. Addressing sensitivity effectively requires a multifaceted approach that encompasses prevention, careful material selection, and technique modifications. This chapter explores these strategies to ensure that minimally invasive treatments not only achieve desired clinical outcomes but also maintain patient comfort and satisfaction.

One of the foundational strategies in managing sensitivity is the prevention of its onset. Prophylactic measures involve both patient education and specific procedural adjustments. Educating patients about the nature of minimally invasive procedures, their benefits, and potential post-treatment sensations can help set realistic expectations and reduce anxiety. Clear communication about what to expect, combined with instructions for post-treatment care, is crucial in minimizing discomfort.

In terms of procedural adjustments, practitioners must consider the impact of their techniques on the tooth structure and surrounding tissues. For instance, when performing procedures such as tooth preparation for veneers or restorations, the depth of enamel removal should be carefully controlled to avoid exposing the underlying dentin, which can increase sensitivity. Additionally, employing gentle techniques and avoiding excessive pressure can prevent unnecessary trauma to the tooth and reduce the risk of sensitivity.

Material selection plays a critical role in managing and preventing sensitivity. The choice of materials for restorations and other dental interventions must be guided by their compatibility with the tooth structure and their ability to protect sensitive areas. For example, when placing composite restorations, the use of low-shrinkage materials and effective bonding agents can minimize the risk of postoperative sensitivity. Moreover, materials that exhibit good thermal insulation properties can help shield the tooth from temperature fluctuations, which are common sources of sensitivity.

Desensitizing agents are another valuable tool in the management of sensitivity. These agents, which include fluoride varnishes, calcium phosphates, and desensitizing pastes, work by occluding dentinal tubules or enhancing the tooth's resistance to external stimuli. Application of these agents can be done both during and after minimally invasive procedures to alleviate sensitivity and promote patient comfort. For instance, fluoride varnishes can be applied to the tooth surface after a procedure to strengthen enamel and reduce the risk of sensitivity.

In cases where sensitivity does arise, prompt and effective

management is essential to prevent long-term discomfort and ensure a positive treatment outcome. For example, patients experiencing sensitivity after a procedure may benefit from using toothpaste formulated for sensitive teeth. These toothpastes contain compounds such as potassium nitrate or strontium chloride, which help to desensitize nerve endings in the dentin and provide relief from discomfort.

Additionally, modifying treatment techniques can help address sensitivity issues as they occur. For example, if a patient reports sensitivity following a filling or bonding procedure, the dentist may need to reassess the occlusion and make necessary adjustments. Ensuring that the restoration is properly contoured and does not interfere with the patient's bite can prevent undue stress on the treated tooth and alleviate sensitivity.

Another important consideration in managing sensitivity is the role of follow-up care. Regular check-ups allow practitioners to monitor the patient's response to treatment and address any emerging issues promptly. This proactive approach helps to identify and resolve sensitivity issues early, contributing to a more favorable overall treatment experience.

In summary, addressing tooth sensitivity in minimally invasive treatments involves a comprehensive approach that includes preventive measures, careful material selection, the use of desensitizing agents, and technique modifications. By employing these strategies, dental professionals can enhance patient comfort and satisfaction while achieving the clinical goals of minimally invasive dentistry. Balancing the benefits of conservative treatment approaches with effective sensitivity management ensures that patients receive the highest standard of care, both in terms of functional outcomes and overall experience.

Managing tooth sensitivity in minimally invasive dentistry requires a nuanced approach that not only addresses the immediate discomfort experienced by patients but also focuses on long-term prevention and patient education. The complexity of sensitivity management lies in its multifactorial nature, where the interplay between dental materials, procedural techniques, and individual patient factors must be carefully balanced to achieve optimal outcomes.

In minimally invasive procedures, where the goal is to preserve as much natural tooth structure as possible, sensitivity can arise from several sources. One common issue is the exposure of dentin, which occurs when procedures, even those designed to be conservative, inadvertently uncover dentinal tubules. These tubules are channels that extend from the tooth's surface to the nerve endings within the dentin, and their exposure can lead to heightened sensitivity to thermal, tactile, or osmotic stimuli.

To mitigate this risk, it is essential for practitioners to use techniques that minimize dentin exposure. For example, during the placement of dental restorations or veneers, careful control of tooth preparation depth can prevent the unnecessary removal of dentin. Additionally, modern adhesive systems and bonding agents play a crucial role in sealing dentinal tubules and protecting the underlying nerve endings. By ensuring that these systems are applied correctly, practitioners can reduce the likelihood of sensitivity post-treatment.

Material selection is another critical factor in the prevention and management of sensitivity. The choice of restorative materials should consider not only their aesthetic and functional properties but also their compatibility with the tooth structure and their impact on patient comfort. For instance, materials with high thermal conductivity can exacerbate sensitivity, while those with insulating properties can help to shield the tooth from temperature changes. Composite resins, when used with effective bonding agents, offer a way to create restorations that are not only durable but also less likely to cause post-operative sensitivity.

Desensitizing agents are an integral part of the sensitivity management toolkit. These agents work by forming a protective barrier over the exposed dentin or by occluding the dentinal tubules to prevent stimuli from reaching the nerve endings. Fluoride varnishes, for example, help to remineralize the tooth surface and reduce sensitivity. Calcium phosphate compounds, such as calcium phosphates and bioactive glass, can also be used to enhance the mineral content of the tooth and provide a buffer against sensitivity.

The application of these agents can be performed during and after the minimally invasive procedure. In some cases, a topical desensitizing agent may be applied directly to the treated area to provide immediate relief. For long-term management, incorporating desensitizing products into the patient's daily oral hygiene routine can offer ongoing protection and comfort.

Technique modifications can also play a significant role in addressing sensitivity. For example, when performing procedures that involve the removal of carious tissue or the placement of restorations, using gentle techniques and avoiding excessive pressure can help to minimize trauma to the tooth and surrounding tissues. Adjustments to occlusion and ensuring that restorations are well-fitted and properly contoured can also prevent undue stress on the treated tooth and reduce sensitivity.

Follow-up care is an essential component of sensitivity management. Regular check-ups allow practitioners to assess the patient's response to treatment and make any necessary adjustments. This proactive approach enables the early identification of sensitivity issues and the implementation of corrective measures before they become more problematic.

Patient education is equally important in managing sensitivity. Educating patients about the potential for sensitivity following minimally invasive procedures and providing clear instructions on how to manage it can help to alleviate concerns and improve overall satisfaction. Patients should be advised on the use of desensitizing toothpastes, the importance of maintaining good oral hygiene, and the need for regular dental visits to monitor their condition.

In conclusion, effectively addressing sensitivity in minimally invasive treatments requires a comprehensive approach that includes preventive measures, careful material selection, the use of desensitizing agents, and technique modifications. By employing these strategies, dental professionals can enhance patient comfort and ensure successful outcomes in minimally invasive dentistry. Balancing the benefits of conservative treatment approaches with effective sensitivity management not only improves patient experience but also supports the overall goals of minimally invasive dental care.

The management of tooth sensitivity in minimally invasive dentistry requires a multi-faceted approach that integrates both immediate and long-term strategies to ensure patient comfort and treatment success. Sensitivity often arises not only due to the procedures themselves but also as a consequence of the materials used and the techniques employed. Understanding and addressing these variables are essential for providing optimal patient care.

One fundamental strategy for managing sensitivity is to use materials and techniques that minimize trauma to the tooth. Advanced dental materials, such as contemporary resin composites and glass ionomer cements, are designed to be more biocompatible and less likely to induce sensitivity compared to older materials. These modern materials often incorporate fluoride-releasing properties or other additives that help to strengthen the tooth structure and reduce the risk of sensitivity.

Resin-based composites, for instance, have improved significantly over the years, providing not only aesthetic benefits but also enhanced adaptation to the tooth structure. The improved bonding agents used with these composites are specifically designed to create a strong bond to both enamel and dentin, which helps to seal the dentinal tubules and prevent sensitivity. Additionally, the use of self-etching adhesives can streamline the bonding process and reduce the potential for post-operative sensitivity by eliminating the need for separate etching and rinsing steps.

In cases where traditional materials and techniques may not be suitable, alternative approaches such as laser therapy or air abrasion can be employed. Laser technology, for example, offers a minimally invasive method to remove carious dentin and prepare tooth surfaces with minimal discomfort. The laser's precision allows for selective removal of diseased tissue while preserving healthy tooth structure, which can help in reducing post-treatment sensitivity. Similarly, air abrasion uses a stream of abrasive particles to prepare the tooth without the heat and vibration associated with traditional drilling, further decreasing the likelihood of sensitivity.

The application of desensitizing agents plays a crucial role in managing sensitivity. These agents work by occluding the dentinal tubules or by forming a protective barrier over the exposed dentin. Fluoride treatments, often used in conjunction with other desensitizing products, enhance the tooth's resistance to demineralization and help to alleviate discomfort. Desensitizing pastes or gels containing potassium nitrate or calcium phosphates can also be beneficial, as they work by either desensitizing the nerve endings within the dentin or promoting remineralization of the tooth structure.

Another aspect of sensitivity management involves the

modification of clinical techniques. Careful control of the depth of preparation and the avoidance of over-preparation are essential to minimize sensitivity. For example, when placing restorations, ensuring that the margins are well-sealed and the restoration is properly contoured can prevent issues such as microleakage or occlusal discrepancies that may lead to sensitivity. Adjusting the occlusion to ensure that the treated tooth does not experience excessive forces during function can also help to alleviate discomfort.

Patient education is a vital component in the management of sensitivity. Patients should be informed about the potential for sensitivity following minimally invasive procedures and advised on how to manage it effectively. This includes recommendations for the use of desensitizing toothpastes, which contain compounds such as potassium nitrate or stannous fluoride that help to reduce sensitivity over time. Patients should also be encouraged to maintain good oral hygiene practices and to avoid overly aggressive brushing, which can exacerbate sensitivity.

In addition to these preventive and therapeutic strategies, regular follow-up visits are important to monitor the patient's response to treatment and to address any ongoing issues. These visits provide an opportunity to assess the effectiveness of the sensitivity management strategies employed and to make any necessary adjustments to the treatment plan.

Ultimately, the goal of managing sensitivity in minimally invasive dentistry is to balance the benefits of conservative treatment approaches with the need for patient comfort and satisfaction. By employing a comprehensive approach that includes careful material selection, effective use of desensitizing agents, modification of techniques, and patient education, dental practitioners can enhance the overall success of minimally invasive procedures and improve patient outcomes.

By addressing sensitivity proactively and thoughtfully, dental professionals can ensure that the advantages of minimally invasive dentistry—such as preserving natural tooth structure and providing aesthetic improvements—are realized without compromising patient comfort. This holistic approach not only enhances the effectiveness of minimally invasive treatments but also supports the long-term success of dental care.

CHAPTER 20: MINIMALLY INVASIVE APPROACHES TO MANAGEMENT OF DENTAL TRAUMA

Dental trauma represents a significant challenge in clinical dentistry, often requiring swift intervention to preserve tooth vitality and function. Minimally invasive approaches to managing dental trauma offer a way to address these injuries conservatively, emphasizing the preservation of natural tooth structure while providing effective treatment. This chapter explores various strategies and techniques for managing traumatic dental injuries with minimal intervention, focusing on the assessment and treatment of fractures, displacements, and other types of trauma.

In managing dental trauma, the primary goal is to assess the extent of the injury and determine the most appropriate intervention to preserve the tooth. The initial evaluation involves a thorough clinical examination combined with radiographic imaging to assess the extent of the trauma, including the presence of fractures, displacements, or other injuries. This diagnostic approach helps in developing a treatment plan tailored to the specific type and severity of the trauma.

For cases involving dental fractures, minimally invasive techniques focus on preserving the remaining tooth structure and restoring function. Enamel and dentin fractures, if confined to the outer layers of the tooth, often require conservative management. Restorative materials such as dental composites can be employed to repair the fractured area while maintaining the tooth's structural integrity and aesthetic appearance. These composite resins are highly adhesive and can be bonded directly to the remaining tooth structure, providing a durable and esthetically pleasing restoration. The use of advanced bonding agents ensures that the composite material adheres well to the tooth surface, minimizing the need for more invasive procedures.

In cases where fractures involve the pulp chamber or extend into the root, the approach may require more detailed consideration. Pulp capping techniques can be used to protect the pulp and encourage its continued vitality. This involves placing a biocompatible material over the exposed pulp to promote healing and prevent further damage. Calcium hydroxide and mineral trioxide aggregate (MTA) are commonly used materials for pulp capping, providing a protective layer while stimulating reparative dentin formation. Minimally invasive pulp capping aims to preserve the vitality of the tooth and prevent the need for more extensive endodontic treatment.

Displaced teeth, such as those that have been luxated or avulsed, also benefit from a minimally invasive approach when managed appropriately. For luxated teeth, the goal is to reposition the tooth into its original socket and stabilize it to facilitate proper healing. This is typically done using gentle, controlled force to avoid further damage to the surrounding tissues. The tooth may be splinted temporarily to maintain its position and allow for natural reattachment to occur.

Modern splinting techniques often use flexible materials that minimize trauma to the surrounding periodontal tissues while providing adequate stabilization.

When managing avulsed teeth, where the tooth has been completely displaced from its socket, the priority is to replant the tooth as soon as possible to maximize the chances of successful reattachment. The avulsed tooth should be handled carefully, ideally by the crown rather than the root, and gently cleaned if necessary before replantation. Storage of the tooth in a suitable medium, such as cold milk or a saline solution, can help to preserve the vitality of the periodontal ligament cells until the tooth can be replanted. Following replantation, the tooth is typically stabilized with a splint for several weeks to support the healing process and prevent further displacement.

In addition to these direct management techniques, minimally invasive approaches also include preventive measures to reduce the risk of future trauma. This may involve the use of protective mouthguards, particularly for patients who participate in contact sports or other high-risk activities. Mouthguards act as a cushion to absorb and distribute impact forces, reducing the likelihood of injury to the teeth and surrounding tissues.

Furthermore, patient education plays a crucial role in minimizing the impact of dental trauma. Educating patients about the importance of prompt treatment following an injury, proper oral hygiene practices, and the use of protective devices can significantly influence the outcome of traumatic dental injuries. Early intervention and adherence to recommended treatments are key factors in preserving tooth vitality and ensuring successful recovery.

Minimally invasive approaches to managing dental trauma prioritize the preservation of natural tooth structure and function, utilizing conservative techniques and materials to address injuries effectively. By employing these strategies, dental professionals can enhance patient outcomes, minimize the need for more invasive procedures, and promote overall dental health.

In the management of dental trauma, the application of minimally invasive techniques emphasizes preserving the natural tooth structure while addressing the immediate concerns of the injury. A comprehensive approach requires understanding the specific type of trauma and employing techniques that not only address the immediate damage but also support long-term tooth vitality and function.

For traumatic dental injuries involving fractures, a critical aspect of minimally invasive management is the assessment of the fracture's extent and its impact on the tooth's vitality. For enamel and dentin fractures, particularly those limited to the outer layers of the tooth, conservative treatments often suffice. The use of adhesive dental materials such as composites allows for the restoration of the tooth's structural and aesthetic integrity. These composites can be sculpted to match the natural contours of the tooth and bonded effectively to the remaining tooth structure, providing a seamless and durable repair.

When fractures extend into the pulp or the root, the approach becomes more complex. In cases where the pulp is exposed or at risk, pulp capping is a viable minimally invasive technique aimed at preserving the tooth's vitality. Materials like calcium hydroxide and mineral trioxide aggregate (MTA) are commonly used in pulp capping procedures. These materials not only protect the pulp but also encourage the formation of secondary dentin, thereby aiding in the tooth's natural healing process. Effective pulp capping minimizes the need for more invasive endodontic treatments and helps maintain the tooth's long-term health.

In situations involving dental displacements, such as luxation or avulsion, the primary objective is to manage the injury while minimizing additional damage. For luxated teeth, where the tooth is displaced but not lost, repositioning the tooth to its original socket and stabilizing it with a splint is crucial. Gentle repositioning minimizes trauma to the surrounding periodontal tissues and helps facilitate natural healing. The splint, often made from flexible materials, supports the tooth while allowing for tissue regeneration and reattachment.

Avulsed teeth present a unique challenge and require prompt intervention. Successful replantation depends on the immediate handling and storage of the avulsed tooth. Ideally, the tooth should be kept moist, with milk or a saline solution being preferable to tap water, which can damage the periodontal ligament cells. Upon replantation, the tooth is stabilized with a splint for a period of weeks to ensure that it remains in place as the surrounding tissues heal and reattach. Post-replantation monitoring is essential to assess the tooth's vitality and detect any potential complications such as root resorption or infection.

In addition to direct management techniques, preventive strategies play a significant role in minimizing the risk and impact of dental trauma. The use of mouthguards, particularly in patients involved in sports or other high-risk activities, can be a highly effective preventive measure. These custom-fitted devices provide a cushion against impact forces, reducing the likelihood of traumatic injuries and preserving the integrity of the teeth and surrounding tissues.

Furthermore, patient education is a vital component of managing dental trauma. Patients should be informed about the importance of timely intervention following an injury, proper oral hygiene practices to prevent complications, and the benefits of protective devices. Educating patients on how to handle avulsed teeth and the importance of immediate dental care can significantly influence the outcome of traumatic dental injuries.

The integration of minimally invasive techniques in managing dental trauma requires a thorough understanding of the injury, careful planning, and execution of conservative treatment strategies. By focusing on preserving natural tooth structure and employing less invasive procedures, dental professionals can enhance patient outcomes and support the long-term health and function of the injured teeth.

Minimally invasive approaches not only aim to address the immediate effects of trauma but also emphasize the importance of ongoing care and monitoring. Regular follow-ups are crucial to assess the success of the treatment, manage any potential complications, and ensure the continued vitality of the affected teeth. This comprehensive approach to dental trauma management underscores the value of preserving natural tooth structure and function, aligning with the principles of minimally invasive dentistry.

In the realm of dental trauma management, the goal of minimally invasive approaches extends beyond the immediate repair of injuries to encompass strategies that promote long-term dental health and function. The following discussion delves deeper into specific techniques and considerations that enhance the management of dental trauma while adhering to the principles of minimal intervention.

When addressing traumatic injuries that involve significant enamel and dentin loss, the use of resin-based composites remains a cornerstone of minimally invasive treatment. These materials offer not only a conservative means to restore the tooth's structure but also provide aesthetic benefits by closely matching the natural tooth color. In situations where the fracture extends into the dentin, careful cavity preparation is essential. This involves the removal of any compromised tissue while preserving as much of the healthy tooth structure as possible. The application of adhesive systems ensures a strong bond between the tooth and the restorative material, which contributes to the durability of the repair and helps prevent future complications.

For cases involving pulp exposure due to trauma, a conservative approach focuses on preserving pulp vitality while addressing the damage. Direct pulp capping, as mentioned earlier, involves placing a protective layer over the exposed pulp to stimulate healing and prevent bacterial infiltration. This technique relies on materials like MTA or calcium hydroxide, which possess properties conducive to pulp preservation and dentin regeneration. In cases where direct pulp capping is not feasible, partial pulpotomy may be employed to remove only the affected portion of the pulp while maintaining the remainder of the pulp tissue. This approach aims to retain the vitality of the pulp and avoid more invasive procedures such as root canal therapy.

Management of dental luxation, where the tooth is displaced but remains in the socket, requires precision in repositioning and stabilization. The initial step involves assessing the degree of displacement and the condition of the supporting periodontal structures. Intraoral radiographs can assist in determining the extent of damage and ensuring that the tooth is properly aligned before stabilization. The application of a flexible splint, often made from composite resin or orthodontic wire, helps maintain the tooth in its proper position while allowing for natural healing. The duration of splinting can vary based on the severity of the luxation and the tooth's response to treatment, with follow-up evaluations necessary to monitor the healing process.

In managing avulsed teeth, the emphasis on prompt and appropriate handling cannot be overstated. After replantation, patients should be monitored closely for signs of root resorption, pulp necrosis, or periodontal issues. The use of calcium hydroxide or antibiotic pastes within the root canal may be considered to manage potential complications and support the tooth's long-term viability. Additionally, long-term follow-up care includes periodic radiographic examinations and clinical assessments to evaluate the health of the tooth and surrounding structures.

Prevention and patient education are integral components of a comprehensive approach to dental trauma. Instructing patients on proper techniques for managing dental injuries, such as how to handle and store an avulsed tooth, can significantly impact treatment outcomes. Providing guidance on the use of mouthguards for sports and other high-risk activities further reduces the likelihood of traumatic injuries and contributes to overall dental health.

Emerging technologies and advancements in dental materials continue to enhance the field of minimally invasive trauma management. Innovations in digital imaging, such as cone-beam computed tomography (CBCT), offer detailed three-dimensional views of traumatic injuries, allowing for more accurate diagnosis and treatment planning. The development of advanced biomaterials, including bioactive glasses and regenerative agents, holds promise for improving the outcomes of conservative treatments and supporting the natural healing processes of dental tissues.

In summary, the application of minimally invasive techniques in the management of dental trauma emphasizes the preservation of natural tooth structure and the promotion of long-term dental health. By employing conservative approaches, utilizing advanced materials, and integrating preventive measures, dental professionals can effectively address traumatic injuries while adhering to the principles of minimal intervention. The continued evolution of dental technologies and materials will further refine these approaches, enhancing the precision, efficacy, and patient comfort in managing dental trauma.

CHAPTER 21: ECONOMIC CONSIDERATIONS IN MINIMALLY INVASIVE DENTISTRY

The economic aspects of adopting minimally invasive dentistry techniques encompass a broad range of considerations that impact both dental practices and patients. This analysis delves into the cost-effectiveness of preventive and conservative treatments, the potential savings associated with reduced need for extensive interventions, and the financial implications for both parties involved. Understanding these economic dimensions is crucial for evaluating the value of minimally invasive practices and their long-term benefits.

At the core of the economic evaluation of minimally invasive dentistry is the comparison between traditional and conservative treatment approaches. Traditional dental care often involves more invasive procedures, such as extensive restorations, root canals, and crowns, which can be costly for both patients and practices. In contrast, minimally invasive techniques focus on prevention and early intervention, aiming to address dental issues before they escalate into more complex conditions. This approach can result in significant cost savings by reducing the frequency and severity of invasive treatments.

One of the primary economic benefits of minimally invasive dentistry is its emphasis on preventive care. Preventive treatments, such as fluoride applications, sealants, and regular dental check-ups, are typically less expensive than restorative procedures. By investing in these preventive measures, dental practices can help patients avoid the need for more costly interventions in the future. Moreover, preventive care can contribute to overall cost savings by reducing the incidence of dental diseases and complications that require expensive treatments.

Another economic advantage of minimally invasive dentistry is the reduction in the need for extensive restorative procedures. Techniques such as microabrasion, conservative fillings, and tooth-colored materials are designed to address dental issues with minimal removal of healthy tooth structure. These approaches not only preserve the natural tooth but also reduce the need for more extensive and expensive restorative work. For example, a small, conservative filling is generally less costly than a full crown or root canal treatment. By minimizing the need for such extensive procedures, dental practices can lower their overall treatment costs and pass on these savings to patients.

The cost-effectiveness of minimally invasive techniques also extends to the management of dental trauma. Conservative approaches to treating traumatic injuries, such as minor fractures or displacements, can often be managed with less invasive procedures and reduced chair time compared to traditional methods. This efficiency can translate into lower treatment costs and increased patient satisfaction. Furthermore, the use of advanced materials and technologies in minimally invasive trauma management can enhance treatment outcomes and reduce the likelihood of complications, which can further contribute to cost savings.

For dental practices, adopting minimally invasive techniques can also impact financial performance. While there may be initial investments in new technologies or materials, these costs are often offset by the benefits of reduced chair time, fewer complications, and increased patient retention. Minimally invasive procedures can streamline workflows, reduce the need for multiple visits, and improve overall practice efficiency. Additionally, by offering preventive and conservative care, dental practices can attract and retain patients who value these approaches, potentially leading to increased patient volume and revenue.

From the patient perspective, the economic implications of minimally invasive dentistry are significant. Patients who receive preventive and conservative treatments may experience lower out-of-pocket costs due to fewer and less extensive procedures. Furthermore, the preservation of natural tooth structure through minimally invasive techniques can reduce the need for more expensive restorative work in the future. The long-term financial benefits of maintaining good oral health and avoiding extensive treatments can be substantial, making minimally invasive dentistry an attractive option for many patients.

In addition to direct cost savings, minimally invasive techniques can also contribute to improved patient outcomes and satisfaction. Patients who experience less discomfort and shorter recovery times may be more likely to adhere to recommended treatment plans and seek regular dental care. This adherence can lead to better oral health outcomes and reduced need for complex treatments, further enhancing the overall economic value of minimally invasive dentistry.

In conclusion, the economic considerations of minimally

invasive dentistry highlight the potential cost savings and financial benefits associated with preventive and conservative approaches. By focusing on early intervention, preserving natural tooth structure, and reducing the need for extensive treatments, minimally invasive techniques offer significant advantages for both dental practices and patients. Understanding these economic dimensions is essential for evaluating the value of minimally invasive practices and their impact on overall dental care costs. As the field continues to evolve, ongoing assessments of economic factors will be crucial in optimizing the delivery of minimally invasive dental care and ensuring its continued success in improving patient outcomes and practice efficiency.

The adoption of minimally invasive dentistry techniques also brings to light various economic implications that extend beyond direct treatment costs. One significant factor in evaluating the economic impact is the potential for reduced overall healthcare costs. Minimally invasive dentistry emphasizes early diagnosis and preventive care, which can avert more complex and expensive dental issues. This proactive approach not only benefits individual patients but also contributes to broader public health savings. For example, managing carious lesions early with conservative treatments can prevent the progression of decay that might otherwise lead to more complex restorations or even tooth loss. By addressing dental problems before they become severe, both healthcare systems and patients can avoid the higher costs associated with advanced dental interventions and related complications.

Additionally, the integration of technology in minimally invasive procedures—such as digital imaging, laser treatments, and advanced diagnostic tools—can contribute to cost-effectiveness in the long term. Although the initial investment in such technologies may be substantial, their use often results in more precise diagnoses, improved treatment outcomes, and reduced need for follow-up visits or re-treatments. For instance, digital impressions and CAD/CAM systems enhance the accuracy of restorations, reducing the likelihood of errors and the need for adjustments or remakes. This precision not only improves patient satisfaction but also streamlines practice workflows, potentially leading to increased productivity and profitability.

From a practice management perspective, minimally invasive techniques can influence revenue generation and patient retention. Offering a range of conservative treatment options can attract patients who are seeking less aggressive dental care, thereby expanding the patient base. Furthermore, the ability to provide effective preventive and conservative treatments can enhance the reputation of a practice, leading to increased referrals and long-term patient loyalty. Practices that invest in minimally invasive technologies and techniques may differentiate themselves in a competitive market, positioning themselves as leaders in modern dental care and improving their market share.

The financial implications for patients, meanwhile, can be considerable. Minimally invasive treatments often result in lower out-of-pocket expenses compared to more extensive procedures. Preventive care, such as routine cleanings and fluoride treatments, typically incurs fewer costs than major restorative work. Additionally, patients who experience fewer complications and require less extensive treatment due to early intervention may benefit from reduced overall dental expenditures. The financial burden of dental care can be a significant concern for many individuals, and the cost-effectiveness of minimally invasive approaches can make quality care more accessible and affordable.

Economic considerations also include the impact on insurance coverage and reimbursement rates. As minimally invasive techniques gain recognition and become more widespread, insurance companies may adjust their coverage policies to reflect the growing emphasis on preventive and conservative care. This shift could potentially lead to changes in reimbursement rates, affecting both dental practices and patients. Practices that adopt minimally invasive approaches may find themselves navigating evolving insurance landscapes and adapting to new reimbursement models that prioritize preventive care.

Moreover, the training and education required to implement minimally invasive techniques can have financial implications for dental professionals. Ongoing professional development and training are necessary to stay current with evolving techniques and technologies. While these investments in education can be significant, they often lead to enhanced skills and the ability to offer advanced treatments, which can ultimately benefit the practice's financial health and patient outcomes.

The overall economic impact of minimally invasive dentistry is multifaceted, involving direct treatment costs, technology investments, patient expenses, and broader healthcare savings. By focusing on prevention and early intervention, minimally invasive approaches offer the potential for significant cost savings and improved financial outcomes for both dental practices and patients. As the field continues to evolve, ongoing evaluation of economic factors will be essential in optimizing the delivery of minimally invasive care and ensuring its sustainability within the dental healthcare system. Embracing these techniques not only aligns with a patient-centered approach to care but also contributes to a more cost-effective and efficient model of dental practice.

In evaluating the economic aspects of minimally invasive dentistry, it is crucial to consider not only the direct and indirect cost savings but also the broader financial implications for the healthcare system. Minimally invasive techniques focus on preserving tooth structure and preventing the escalation of dental issues, which can translate into significant long-term economic benefits.

One of the primary advantages of minimally invasive dentistry is its potential for reducing the overall cost of dental care. By prioritizing prevention and early intervention, these techniques often mitigate the need for more complex and costly treatments. For instance, early detection and management of carious lesions through preventive measures and conservative treatments can avert the progression of decay that might otherwise require extensive restorative procedures. This approach not only saves on the direct costs associated with advanced treatments but also reduces the potential for secondary complications that could further escalate expenses.

The economic impact extends beyond individual patient care to influence public health expenditures. Preventive and minimally invasive treatments help to alleviate the burden on public health systems by reducing the prevalence of severe dental conditions that require costly interventions. By promoting early diagnosis and conservative management, healthcare systems can achieve significant cost savings and improve overall dental health outcomes at a population level.

From a practice management perspective, the adoption of minimally invasive techniques can lead to increased operational efficiency and profitability. The implementation of advanced technologies, such as digital imaging and CAD/CAM systems, may initially require substantial investment. However, these technologies enhance diagnostic accuracy and treatment precision, leading to fewer procedural errors and reduced need for follow-up treatments. As a result, practices can benefit from streamlined workflows, higher patient throughput, and improved financial performance.

Furthermore, minimally invasive dentistry aligns with a patient-centered care model, which can positively impact patient satisfaction and retention. Patients who receive conservative, less invasive treatments often experience less discomfort and faster recovery times, leading to higher levels of satisfaction and loyalty. This, in turn, can contribute to a practice's financial stability by fostering positive patient experiences and encouraging repeat visits and referrals.

Economic considerations also include the potential impact on insurance reimbursement and coverage. As the emphasis on preventive and minimally invasive care grows, insurance providers may adjust their coverage policies to reflect these changes. Practices that offer minimally invasive treatments may need to navigate evolving reimbursement models and negotiate with insurers to ensure adequate compensation for their services. This ongoing dialogue between dental practices and insurance companies will be essential in addressing the financial aspects of minimally invasive care.

Training and education costs are another economic factor to consider. The integration of minimally invasive techniques often requires dental professionals to undergo additional training and certification. While these investments in professional development can be significant, they are essential for ensuring that practitioners are proficient in the latest techniques and technologies. Over time, the benefits of enhanced skills and expertise can outweigh the initial costs, contributing to improved patient outcomes and increased practice revenue.

In addition to the financial implications for dental practices and patients, minimally invasive dentistry can influence broader economic trends within the healthcare sector. The shift towards preventive and conservative care reflects a growing emphasis on cost-effectiveness and value-based healthcare. By adopting these approaches, dental practices contribute to a more sustainable and efficient model of care that prioritizes long-term health outcomes and cost savings.

Ultimately, the economic benefits of minimally invasive dentistry are multifaceted and encompass a range of factors, including reduced treatment costs, increased practice efficiency, improved patient satisfaction, and potential changes in insurance reimbursement. As the field continues to evolve, ongoing analysis of these economic aspects will be crucial in optimizing the delivery of minimally invasive care and ensuring its sustainability within the broader healthcare system. By embracing these techniques, dental professionals can enhance the quality of care they provide while contributing to a more cost-effective and patient-centered approach to dental health.

CHAPTER 22: MINIMALLY INVASIVE TECHNIQUES FOR PEDIATRIC DENTISTRY

In the realm of pediatric dentistry, the application of minimally invasive techniques offers a nuanced approach tailored specifically to the needs of young patients. This chapter delves into how these techniques are adapted for children, emphasizing preventive care, conservative restorations, and strategies designed to address the unique challenges associated with treating this age group.

Minimally invasive techniques in pediatric dentistry prioritize the preservation of natural tooth structure while managing dental issues in a manner that is both effective and considerate of a child's developmental stage. At the heart of these techniques is a commitment to early intervention and preventive care, which aligns with the broader goals of minimizing the extent of treatment needed over a child's lifetime.

Preventive care is fundamental in pediatric dentistry and serves as the cornerstone of minimally invasive practices. Regular check-ups and dental cleanings are essential in identifying potential issues before they progress. Techniques such as fluoride varnishes and dental sealants play a critical role in this preventive strategy. Fluoride varnishes, for example, help in remineralizing early carious lesions, effectively halting their progression without the need for more invasive procedures. Dental sealants, applied to the chewing surfaces of molars, create a protective barrier that shields the enamel from decay-causing bacteria and acids.

The emphasis on conservative restorations in pediatric dentistry reflects the principle of preserving as much natural tooth structure as possible. When a cavity does develop, the approach typically involves techniques that limit the extent of the intervention. For instance, the use of atraumatic restorative treatment (ART) is particularly well-suited for young patients. ART involves the removal of decayed tissue using hand instruments rather than rotary drills, followed by the application of a restorative material. This method minimizes discomfort and stress for the child, which is crucial given their often heightened sensitivity to dental procedures.

Another technique that exemplifies the minimally invasive approach in pediatric dentistry is the use of resin-based composite materials for restorations. These materials not only blend aesthetically with natural tooth structure but also require less tooth preparation compared to traditional amalgam fillings. This reduced need for tooth removal is beneficial in maintaining the integrity of the tooth and minimizing the potential for future dental issues.

Behavior management is a key component of pediatric dentistry that intersects with the principles of minimally invasive care. Techniques designed to improve a child's comfort and cooperation during dental visits are essential for the successful implementation of conservative treatments. Strategies such as tell-show-do, where the dentist explains and demonstrates procedures in a non-threatening manner, can help in reducing anxiety and improving the child's experience. Additionally, creating a positive and welcoming environment in the dental office, with child-friendly decor and engaging activities, contributes to a more relaxed atmosphere that supports minimally invasive techniques.

Pediatric dentists must also navigate the challenges associated with treating young patients who may have difficulty understanding and following oral hygiene instructions. In these cases, education and parental involvement are crucial. Dentists often work closely with parents to establish effective home care routines and address any issues related to diet and oral hygiene. This collaborative approach ensures that preventive measures are reinforced outside the dental office, enhancing the effectiveness of minimally invasive treatments.

The role of minimally invasive techniques extends beyond routine care and into the management of specific conditions that are prevalent among children. For instance, managing early childhood caries (ECC) requires a particularly sensitive approach due to the rapid progression of decay in young children. Minimally invasive techniques such as silver diamine fluoride (SDF) have shown promise in arresting carious lesions in ECC cases. SDF acts as both a preventive and therapeutic agent, effectively halting the progression of decay while being gentle enough to use on young patients.

In addition to these preventive and restorative techniques, the integration of digital technologies into pediatric dentistry also enhances the minimally invasive approach. Digital imaging, for example, offers a less intrusive means of diagnosing and monitoring dental issues compared to traditional radiography. This technology allows for more accurate assessments of dental health and aids in planning minimally invasive treatments with greater precision.

In conclusion, the application of minimally invasive

techniques in pediatric dentistry reflects a comprehensive approach to managing the unique needs of young patients. By emphasizing preventive care, conservative restorations, and effective behavior management, pediatric dentists can provide high-quality care that prioritizes the preservation of natural tooth structure and promotes long-term dental health. These techniques not only address immediate dental issues but also lay the foundation for a positive dental experience and healthy oral habits that will benefit children throughout their lives.

In pediatric dentistry, the application of minimally invasive techniques requires a delicate balance between effective treatment and the preservation of natural tooth structure, tailored specifically to the unique needs and behavioral traits of young patients. This approach not only addresses immediate dental concerns but also fosters long-term oral health through preventive care and conservative management strategies.

A significant aspect of minimally invasive pediatric dentistry is the adoption of advanced diagnostic and preventive tools that allow for early detection and intervention. The use of high-resolution digital imaging techniques, such as intraoral cameras and digital X-rays, has revolutionized the way pediatric dentists assess and monitor dental health. These technologies provide detailed, real-time images that enable the early identification of issues such as incipient carious lesions or developmental anomalies, which might otherwise go unnoticed with traditional methods. The precision offered by these tools supports a proactive approach to dental care, allowing for timely and less invasive treatments.

Fluoride treatments continue to be a cornerstone in the preventive care of children's teeth. The application of fluoride varnishes is particularly effective in strengthening enamel and making it more resistant to decay. Unlike traditional fluoride gels, varnishes can be applied quickly and easily, and they adhere well to the tooth surface, providing extended protection against carious lesions. This technique is highly beneficial in pediatric dentistry, where frequent applications can help combat the high risk of caries often seen in young patients.

The integration of sealants into a child's preventive regimen is another example of minimally invasive care. Dental sealants are thin, protective coatings applied to the chewing surfaces of molars, where pits and fissures can trap food and bacteria, leading to decay. Sealants act as a barrier, preventing bacteria and acids from reaching the tooth enamel. They are particularly effective in pediatric patients due to their propensity for caries in the occlusal surfaces of newly erupted molars. The application process is quick and non-invasive, making it well-suited for children who may be apprehensive about more involved procedures.

Conservative restorative techniques are central to the minimally invasive philosophy in pediatric dentistry. The goal is to address dental issues while preserving as much of the natural tooth structure as possible. For instance, when managing early carious lesions, pediatric dentists often use methods like the ART (Atraumatic Restorative Treatment). This technique involves the removal of carious dentin using hand instruments rather than mechanical drills, followed by the placement of a restorative material. This approach minimizes discomfort and reduces the need for extensive tooth preparation, which is particularly advantageous for treating young children who may have a lower tolerance for dental procedures.

Another promising technique is the use of resin infiltration, which is a minimally invasive method for managing early carious lesions. Resin infiltration involves applying a low-viscosity resin into the porous structure of an incipient carious lesion. This technique effectively halts the progression of caries by sealing the lesion and reinforcing the tooth structure without the need for traditional drilling. Resin infiltration is especially useful in treating carious lesions in anterior teeth, where preserving tooth aesthetics is crucial.

Behavior management techniques are integral to the successful implementation of minimally invasive treatments in pediatric dentistry. Creating a positive dental experience is essential for ensuring that children remain cooperative and comfortable during their visits. Techniques such as positive reinforcement, distraction, and the use of child-friendly language help in reducing anxiety and improving the child's overall experience. Establishing a rapport with young patients and their families also contributes to better outcomes, as it fosters trust and encourages adherence to recommended preventive measures and treatment plans.

In addition to behavioral strategies, technological advancements have further enhanced the effectiveness of minimally invasive techniques in pediatric dentistry. Laser technology, for example, offers a non-invasive alternative for treating early carious lesions and performing soft tissue procedures. Laser systems can be used for caries removal, tissue contouring, and even frenectomies with minimal discomfort and reduced bleeding. The precision of lasers and their ability to promote faster healing make them an attractive option for managing dental issues in young patients.

Overall, the application of minimally invasive techniques in pediatric dentistry represents a forward-thinking approach that prioritizes the preservation of natural tooth structure and the comfort of young patients. By leveraging advanced diagnostic tools, preventive measures, and conservative restorative methods, pediatric dentists can effectively address dental issues while minimizing the need for more invasive procedures. This holistic approach not only improves immediate dental health but also sets the foundation for a lifetime of positive oral health experiences.

In advancing minimally invasive techniques for pediatric dentistry, the focus extends beyond the immediate treatment of dental issues to include a broader perspective on long-term oral health management and behavior modification. This emphasis on a comprehensive approach is critical in managing young patients, who require tailored care strategies that align with their developmental stages and psychological needs.

One of the core principles of minimally invasive pediatric dentistry is the early detection and intervention of dental problems. Early diagnosis, facilitated by modern diagnostic technologies, allows for interventions that are less disruptive and more effective. For example, the use of digital radiography in pediatric settings provides a clear view of tooth and bone structure with minimal radiation exposure. This technology supports the detection of carious lesions at their earliest stages, allowing for preventative or minimally invasive treatments that can significantly alter the trajectory of a child's dental health.

Fluoride treatments remain central to preventive strategies in pediatric dentistry. The application of fluoride varnishes, for instance, has been shown to effectively strengthen enamel and reduce the incidence of caries. These varnishes offer the advantage of easy application and prolonged fluoride release, making them particularly suitable for children who may have difficulty adhering to more complex oral hygiene practices. The use of fluoride gels and foams, while still valuable, are often used in combination with varnishes to provide comprehensive protection against decay.

Sealants, another fundamental preventive measure, play a crucial role in protecting the occlusal surfaces of molars from carious lesions. The process of sealant application involves a simple and painless procedure that is well-received by children. Sealants create a protective barrier over the grooves and pits in the molars, which are prone to decay due to their complex anatomy. By sealing these areas, pediatric dentists can prevent the development of cavities and maintain the integrity of the tooth structure.

Restorative treatments in pediatric dentistry must be approached with sensitivity to the child's comfort and emotional state. Techniques such as minimally invasive restorations aim to address carious lesions while preserving as much healthy tooth structure as possible. Resin-based composites, for example, offer an effective solution for restoring teeth affected by caries without the need for extensive tooth removal. These materials are bonded to the tooth structure, providing a durable and aesthetic result that is particularly important in visible areas such as anterior teeth.

Atraumatic restorative treatment (ART) is another technique that exemplifies the minimally invasive philosophy. ART involves the removal of carious tissue using hand instruments, followed by the placement of a filling material. This approach eliminates the need for mechanical drilling, reducing discomfort and the risk of anxiety in young patients. ART is particularly beneficial in treating early childhood caries, a condition that affects many young children and requires a careful, conservative approach to treatment.

In addition to these techniques, the management of dental trauma in children is an important aspect of pediatric care. Minimally invasive approaches to dental trauma focus on preserving tooth vitality and minimizing further damage. For example, in cases of traumatic dental injuries such as fractures or displacements, techniques such as repositioning and stabilization of the affected tooth can be performed with minimal intervention. The use of dental splints to stabilize mobile teeth or the application of composite resins to restore fractured teeth are examples of conservative strategies that prioritize the preservation of natural tooth structure.

Behavior management is a key component of successful minimally invasive pediatric dentistry. Techniques to help children cope with dental procedures and reduce anxiety are essential for achieving positive outcomes. Strategies such as the use of distraction techniques, including visual and auditory aids, can help divert the child's attention away from the procedure and create a more relaxed environment. Additionally, the use of positive reinforcement and child-friendly communication helps build trust and encourages cooperation, making the dental experience more pleasant and less stressful.

The integration of laser technology into pediatric dentistry offers a modern approach to many of these challenges. Lasers provide a precise and minimally invasive option for various procedures, including caries removal and soft tissue management. The use of lasers can reduce the need for traditional drills and associated noise, which can be particularly distressing for young patients. Furthermore, lasers can promote faster healing and reduce the risk of post-treatment discomfort, contributing to a more positive overall experience for children.

In conclusion, the application of minimally invasive techniques in pediatric dentistry represents a progressive shift towards a more patient-centered and preventative approach to oral health care. By focusing on early detection, conservative treatment methods, and effective behavior management, pediatric dentists can address dental issues with greater precision and less discomfort. This approach not only enhances the immediate care of young patients but also sets the foundation for a lifetime of healthy dental habits and positive dental experiences.

CHAPTER 23: EVIDENCE-BASED PRACTICE IN MINIMALLY INVASIVE DENTISTRY

The integration of evidence-based practice into minimally invasive dentistry represents a critical advancement in the pursuit of optimal patient outcomes and effective clinical strategies. Evidence-based dentistry (EBD) is a paradigm that emphasizes the use of the best available research evidence to inform clinical decision-making, ensuring that patient care is grounded in robust scientific data rather than anecdote or tradition.

Central to evidence-based practice is the rigorous evaluation of clinical research and its application to real-world settings. In minimally invasive dentistry, this involves scrutinizing studies that assess the efficacy and safety of various techniques and materials. For practitioners, the process begins with the identification of pertinent research questions and the gathering of high-quality evidence from systematic reviews, randomized controlled trials, and other credible sources. By focusing on these rigorous study designs, clinicians can ensure that their practices are supported by the most reliable and current evidence available.

The application of evidence-based principles to minimally invasive techniques involves several key steps. First, clinicians must critically appraise the quality of research evidence. This involves evaluating the methodology of studies, including the study design, sample size, statistical analysis, and potential biases. High-quality evidence typically comes from well-conducted randomized controlled trials (RCTs) or systematic reviews that aggregate findings from multiple studies. These types of research provide a higher level of confidence in the validity of the results and their applicability to clinical practice.

Second, evidence must be interpreted in the context of individual patient needs and preferences. While scientific evidence provides a foundation for clinical decisions, patient-centered care requires consideration of each patient's unique situation, including their oral health status, risk factors, and personal preferences. For instance, while evidence may support the use of certain conservative restorative materials, the choice of material for a specific patient may also depend on factors such as aesthetic considerations, cost, and patient comfort. Thus, evidence-based practice requires a balance between scientific evidence and individualized patient care.

One important area of focus in minimally invasive dentistry is the evaluation of new technologies and techniques. For example, the use of laser technology in dental treatments is a relatively recent innovation. Evidence-based practice involves assessing clinical trials and systematic reviews that examine the efficacy of lasers for various procedures, such as caries removal or soft tissue management. By analyzing outcomes such as treatment success rates, patient comfort, and procedural efficiency, clinicians can determine whether laser technology offers tangible benefits over traditional methods and how it can be best integrated into clinical practice.

The field of minimally invasive dentistry also benefits from evidence-based approaches to preventive care. For instance, the effectiveness of fluoride treatments, dental sealants, and dietary counseling in preventing caries is well-documented in scientific literature. Evidence-based guidelines for these preventive measures help clinicians develop treatment protocols that are both effective and efficient. By adhering to guidelines supported by strong evidence, dental practitioners can optimize preventive care strategies and reduce the incidence of carious lesions and other oral health issues.

Moreover, evidence-based practice plays a crucial role in the ongoing development of treatment protocols. As new research emerges, it is essential for dental professionals to stay informed about the latest findings and integrate them into their practice. Continuing education and professional development are integral to maintaining an evidence-based approach. Regular review of current literature, participation in professional networks, and engagement with clinical guidelines ensure that practitioners remain up-to-date with the latest advancements and best practices in minimally invasive dentistry.

The dissemination of evidence-based knowledge also involves the translation of research findings into practical recommendations and clinical guidelines. Organizations such as the American Dental Association (ADA) and the Cochrane Collaboration produce guidelines and systematic reviews that synthesize research evidence and provide actionable recommendations for clinicians. These resources are invaluable for dental practitioners seeking to implement evidence-based practices and improve patient outcomes.

In summary, evidence-based practice in minimally invasive dentistry underscores the importance of integrating scientific research with clinical expertise and patient preferences.

By focusing on high-quality evidence and applying it to individual patient care, dental practitioners can enhance the efficacy of minimally invasive techniques and promote optimal oral health outcomes. This approach not only fosters the advancement of dental practice but also ensures that patient care is informed by the most reliable and current evidence available. The commitment to evidence-based practice ultimately leads to more effective treatments, improved patient satisfaction, and the continued evolution of minimally invasive dentistry.

The transition from traditional dental practices to evidence-based minimally invasive techniques necessitates a comprehensive understanding of how clinical research informs treatment decisions. This approach ensures that practices are not only grounded in scientific evidence but also align with the latest advancements in dental care.

One crucial aspect of evidence-based practice is the systematic review of literature that provides insights into the efficacy of various minimally invasive techniques. Systematic reviews aggregate data from multiple studies, offering a comprehensive evaluation of treatment outcomes. For example, systematic reviews of adhesive materials and techniques can reveal their effectiveness in different clinical scenarios, such as their longevity, bond strength, and resistance to failure. Such reviews enable practitioners to make informed decisions based on a synthesis of high-quality evidence rather than isolated studies.

In addition to systematic reviews, meta-analyses play a vital role in evidence-based practice. Meta-analyses use statistical methods to combine data from several studies, enhancing the precision of effect estimates. This is particularly useful in assessing the efficacy of new technologies or treatment modalities in minimally invasive dentistry. For instance, a meta-analysis of laser treatments for caries removal can provide a clearer picture of their effectiveness compared to traditional methods, taking into account various factors such as treatment duration, patient comfort, and success rates.

Critical appraisal of individual studies is also fundamental to evidence-based practice. Clinicians must assess the methodological quality of research to determine the reliability and applicability of the findings. Key factors in this appraisal include the study design, sample size, control measures, and statistical analyses. For instance, well-designed randomized controlled trials (RCTs) with robust sample sizes and appropriate controls are generally considered the gold standard in clinical research. However, even observational studies and cohort studies can provide valuable insights, especially when RCTs are not feasible.

Another important consideration is the relevance of research findings to the specific clinical context. Evidence-based practice requires clinicians to evaluate how research outcomes apply to their patient population and clinical setting. For example, while studies may show that a particular minimally invasive technique is effective in a research setting, its application in everyday practice may differ. Factors such as patient demographics, local resources, and practice settings must be considered to ensure that evidence-based recommendations are practical and beneficial for the patients being treated.

The integration of evidence-based techniques into clinical practice also involves the development and use of clinical guidelines. These guidelines, often produced by professional organizations or expert panels, offer practical recommendations based on a thorough review of the evidence. For minimally invasive dentistry, guidelines may address a range of topics, from the appropriate use of fluoride and sealants to the application of new adhesive technologies and caries management strategies. Adhering to these guidelines helps ensure that treatments are consistent with the latest evidence and best practices.

Educational initiatives and professional development play a significant role in promoting evidence-based practice. Continuing education programs, workshops, and conferences provide opportunities for dental professionals to stay updated on the latest research and advancements. Engaging with these educational resources helps practitioners integrate new evidence into their practice and refine their clinical skills. Additionally, participation in research activities and collaborations with academic institutions can further enhance a clinician's ability to apply evidence-based practices effectively.

The patient's perspective is also an essential component of evidence-based practice. Effective communication between clinician and patient ensures that treatment decisions are made collaboratively, considering both scientific evidence and patient preferences. For example, when discussing treatment options for carious lesions, a clinician might present evidence on the effectiveness of various minimally invasive techniques, such as fluoride varnishes or resin infiltration, while also addressing the patient's concerns and preferences. This approach fosters shared decision-making and enhances patient satisfaction.

The role of evidence-based practice in minimally invasive dentistry extends beyond individual treatments to encompass overall practice management. By adopting evidence-based approaches, dental practices can improve their efficiency, reduce costs, and enhance patient outcomes. For instance, evidence-based preventive strategies, such as routine use of sealants and fluoride treatments, can reduce the incidence of caries and subsequently lower the need for more extensive restorative procedures. This not only benefits patients by preserving tooth structure but also helps practices optimize their resource allocation and operational efficiency.

In conclusion, the evidence-based approach to minimally invasive dentistry is integral to advancing dental practice and improving patient care. By systematically evaluating and applying research evidence, clinicians can enhance the effectiveness of minimally invasive techniques, ensure patient-centered care, and contribute to the overall progress of dental science. The commitment to evidence-based practice requires ongoing education, critical appraisal of research, and a focus on integrating scientific findings with clinical expertise and patient preferences. This approach not only fosters better clinical outcomes but also upholds the principles of quality and excellence in dental care.

In advancing evidence-based practice within minimally invasive dentistry, it is essential to address how clinicians can translate research findings into practical applications. This involves not only understanding the research but also implementing it in a way that is feasible and beneficial in everyday clinical settings.

One key aspect of integrating evidence into practice is the use of decision-support tools and resources. These tools can assist practitioners in applying the latest research findings to their clinical decision-making processes. For example, clinical decision support systems (CDSS) can provide real-time access to evidence-based guidelines and recommendations during patient consultations. By leveraging these systems, practitioners can ensure that their decisions are aligned with the most current evidence, enhancing the accuracy and effectiveness of their treatments.

The application of evidence-based practices also requires a thorough understanding of how to evaluate the quality and relevance of research. It is crucial for clinicians to be adept at distinguishing between high-quality evidence and studies with potential biases or limitations. This involves assessing the study design, sample size, statistical methods, and potential conflicts of interest. For instance, while randomized controlled trials (RCTs) are often considered the gold standard, other types of research, such as cohort studies or case-control studies, can still offer valuable insights, particularly when RCTs are not practical or ethical.

Another important factor in implementing evidence-based practices is the continuous monitoring and evaluation of outcomes. Clinicians should regularly review patient outcomes and treatment effectiveness to ensure that the adopted techniques are yielding the desired results. This ongoing evaluation helps identify areas for improvement and provides feedback for refining clinical practices. For example, tracking the success rates of different minimally invasive techniques, such as resin infiltration or selective carious dentin removal, can inform future treatment decisions and contribute to the overall enhancement of care quality.

Patient education and involvement are integral to the evidence-based approach. Educating patients about the benefits and limitations of various minimally invasive techniques empowers them to make informed decisions about their treatment options. Providing patients with clear, evidence-based information helps build trust and facilitates shared decision-making. For example, when discussing options for managing early carious lesions, presenting evidence on the efficacy of fluoride treatments compared to more invasive restorative procedures allows patients to weigh the benefits and make choices that align with their preferences and values.

The integration of evidence-based practices into clinical workflows also requires effective communication and collaboration among dental team members. Ensuring that all team members are aware of and adhere to evidence-based guidelines promotes consistency in patient care. Regular team meetings, training sessions, and updates on recent research developments can facilitate this collaboration. Additionally, fostering a culture of continuous learning and improvement within the dental practice supports the ongoing integration of evidence-based techniques.

The impact of evidence-based practice extends beyond individual patient care to influence broader aspects of dental practice management. By adopting evidence-based preventive strategies and treatments, practices can optimize their resource utilization and reduce the overall cost of care. For example, investing in preventive measures that have been shown to be effective in reducing caries incidence can ultimately lower the need for more costly restorative procedures. This not only benefits patients by minimizing the extent of their dental interventions but also enhances the financial sustainability of dental practices.

Furthermore, evidence-based practice plays a crucial role in advancing the field of minimally invasive dentistry through research and innovation. By participating in and supporting clinical research, practitioners contribute to the generation of new knowledge and the refinement of existing techniques. This collaborative approach to research and practice fosters a dynamic environment where evidence-based practices can continually evolve and improve.

In conclusion, the successful implementation of evidence-based practices in minimally invasive dentistry relies on a multifaceted approach that includes evaluating research quality, utilizing decision-support tools, continuously monitoring outcomes, and involving patients in their care. By integrating the latest scientific evidence into clinical practice, dental professionals can enhance the effectiveness of minimally invasive techniques, improve patient outcomes, and contribute to the ongoing advancement of dental care. This commitment to evidence-based practice not only upholds the highest standards of care but also ensures that dental practices remain at the forefront of innovation and excellence in the field.

CHAPTER 24: INTEGRATING MINIMALLY INVASIVE TECHNIQUES WITH TRADITIONAL METHODS

In the evolving landscape of dental practice, the integration of minimally invasive techniques with traditional methods represents a crucial advancement. This chapter aims to elucidate the synergy between these two approaches, demonstrating how their combination can enhance patient care, address complex clinical scenarios, and optimize treatment outcomes. By examining the integration of minimally invasive techniques with established methods, we gain insights into how these modalities can complement each other, leading to more effective and comprehensive dental care.

Minimally invasive dentistry focuses on preserving as much of the natural tooth structure as possible while employing techniques that are less traumatic and more conservative. Traditional dental methods, on the other hand, often involve more extensive procedures and restorations. The challenge and opportunity lie in harmonizing these approaches to leverage the strengths of both. This integration requires a nuanced understanding of when and how to employ each technique to maximize patient benefit.

One of the foundational aspects of integrating minimally invasive and traditional techniques is the evaluation of the clinical situation. This begins with a comprehensive assessment of the patient's oral health, including diagnostic imaging and clinical examination. For instance, in cases of extensive carious lesions or complex restorations, a traditional approach may initially seem more appropriate due to its well-established protocols for managing severe cases. However, incorporating minimally invasive techniques, such as caries removal using laser or air abrasion methods, can often reduce the extent of intervention needed, thereby preserving more healthy tooth structure and enhancing patient comfort.

The use of minimally invasive techniques in conjunction with traditional methods can be particularly advantageous in the management of complex dental conditions. Consider, for example, the treatment of a tooth with significant carious involvement and associated structural damage. A traditional approach might involve extensive drilling and restoration. However, by integrating minimally invasive techniques such as selective carious dentin removal and the application of advanced bonding agents, practitioners can reduce the amount of tooth structure lost while still effectively addressing the carious lesions. This hybrid approach not only helps in maintaining tooth vitality but also improves the long-term prognosis of the restoration.

Another critical area where integration plays a vital role is in the management of periodontal conditions. Traditional periodontal treatments often involve scaling and root planing, which can be complemented by minimally invasive techniques such as laser therapy. Laser technology offers precision in soft tissue management, reduces patient discomfort, and accelerates healing. Combining laser treatment with conventional periodontal therapies allows for a more comprehensive approach, addressing both the microbial factors and the soft tissue health of the periodontium. This integrated strategy can lead to better outcomes and more efficient management of periodontal disease.

In restorative dentistry, the integration of minimally invasive techniques with traditional methods can enhance the overall treatment strategy. For example, when placing dental crowns or veneers, minimally invasive techniques such as digital impressions and adhesive bonding can be combined with traditional crown preparation. Digital impressions offer improved accuracy and patient comfort compared to traditional mold-taking methods, while adhesive bonding ensures a strong, durable connection between the tooth and the restoration. By integrating these techniques, clinicians can provide restorations that are both functionally effective and aesthetically pleasing.

The integration of minimally invasive and traditional approaches also extends to preventive care. Traditional preventive measures, such as fluoride treatments and sealants, can be augmented with minimally invasive techniques like resin infiltration for the management of incipient carious lesions. Resin infiltration, which involves the application of a low-viscosity resin to early carious lesions, helps to halt the progression of caries without the need for more invasive procedures. Combining this with traditional preventive strategies enhances the effectiveness of caries management and supports overall oral health.

Effective integration requires careful planning and execution. Clinicians must be adept at assessing which techniques will offer the best outcomes based on the specific clinical scenario and patient needs. This often involves a thorough understanding of the strengths and limitations of both minimally invasive and traditional methods. Continuing education and training in both areas are essential for staying current with advancements and ensuring that the integration of these approaches is both safe and effective.

Moreover, patient communication plays a crucial role in the integration process. Patients need to be informed about the benefits and limitations of both minimally invasive and traditional techniques. By providing clear explanations and discussing the rationale behind the chosen treatment plan, practitioners can help patients make informed decisions and feel more confident in their care. This collaborative approach not only improves patient satisfaction but also fosters a stronger therapeutic relationship.

In conclusion, the integration of minimally invasive techniques with traditional methods represents a significant advancement in dental practice. By combining these approaches, practitioners can enhance patient care, address complex cases more effectively, and achieve better outcomes. This integration requires a thorough understanding of both techniques, careful planning, and effective patient communication. As dental practices continue to evolve, the ability to seamlessly blend minimally invasive and traditional methods will remain a key factor in providing comprehensive, high-quality care.

The integration of minimally invasive techniques with traditional methods in dentistry is not merely a juxtaposition of approaches but rather a sophisticated synthesis that leverages the strengths of both to provide superior patient care. This approach necessitates an understanding of the distinct advantages and limitations inherent in each method and the ability to harmonize them effectively within the clinical setting.

One critical area where integration proves beneficial is in

the management of carious lesions. Traditionally, caries management often involved significant removal of tooth structure to ensure that all carious tissue was eradicated before placing restorative materials. While this approach aimed to ensure the longevity of the restoration, it sometimes led to unnecessary loss of healthy tooth structure. Minimally invasive techniques, such as air abrasion and laser therapy, offer a less invasive alternative for caries removal, which can be integrated with traditional restorative methods. For instance, after using a laser to remove carious dentin, a dentist might proceed with traditional methods of cavity preparation and restoration. This combination allows for the preservation of more tooth structure while still ensuring the effective treatment of carious lesions.

Similarly, in restorative dentistry, integrating minimally invasive techniques with traditional methods can enhance outcomes and patient satisfaction. Consider the process of placing a dental crown. Traditionally, crown preparation involved extensive removal of tooth structure to create a suitable abutment. With the advent of minimally invasive techniques such as digital impressions and improved adhesive systems, the process has become more conservative. Digital impressions eliminate the need for traditional mold-taking, which can be uncomfortable for patients and sometimes less accurate. The use of advanced adhesive systems reduces the need for extensive tooth reduction, as these systems can bond effectively to the tooth structure. Integrating these techniques with traditional crown preparation allows for a more comfortable patient experience and potentially better clinical results.

The integration of minimally invasive techniques also extends to the management of periodontal conditions. Traditional periodontal therapy often involves mechanical debridement of the root surfaces to remove plaque and calculus, which can sometimes be invasive and cause discomfort. By incorporating laser therapy into the treatment plan, clinicians can achieve more precise decontamination of the periodontal tissues with less trauma to the patient. Laser therapy can be used alongside traditional scaling and root planing to enhance the treatment of periodontal disease. This combination allows for a more comprehensive approach that addresses both the microbial load and the health of the soft tissue, potentially leading to improved clinical outcomes.

In complex cases involving trauma or significant structural damage, the integration of minimally invasive techniques with traditional methods can provide a more comprehensive treatment plan. For example, in managing a fractured tooth, a traditional approach might involve significant restorative work to repair the damage. However, minimally invasive techniques such as direct composite restorations can be used to address smaller fractures or to build up the tooth before applying traditional crowns or other restorations. This strategy not only helps in preserving tooth structure but also optimizes the overall treatment approach by combining the strengths of both methods.

Patient-centered care is another crucial aspect of integrating minimally invasive techniques with traditional methods. Effective communication with patients about their treatment options, including the benefits and limitations of both approaches, is essential for informed decision-making. Patients should be educated about how integrating these techniques can offer more conservative, effective, and comfortable treatment options. By fostering a collaborative relationship with patients, dentists can ensure that treatment plans are tailored to individual needs and preferences, enhancing patient satisfaction and compliance.

Moreover, the integration of these techniques requires ongoing professional development and familiarity with the latest advancements in both minimally invasive and traditional methods. Dentists must stay informed about new technologies, materials, and techniques to effectively combine these approaches. Continuing education and training are essential for mastering the integration process and for ensuring that both minimally invasive and traditional methods are used to their fullest potential.

Ultimately, the successful integration of minimally invasive techniques with traditional methods hinges on the ability to evaluate each clinical situation comprehensively and to apply the most appropriate techniques accordingly. This approach not only aims to achieve the best possible outcomes for patients but also seeks to enhance the overall quality of dental care. As the field of dentistry continues to evolve, the ability to seamlessly blend minimally invasive and traditional methods will remain a cornerstone of providing high-quality, patient-centered care. This integration ensures that patients receive the benefits of both approaches, leading to improved clinical results and enhanced overall dental health.

In addressing the practical application of integrating minimally invasive techniques with traditional methods, it is essential to recognize the value that each approach brings to the table. This integration is not simply a matter of employing different techniques in isolation but involves a strategic amalgamation of approaches to optimize patient outcomes and improve the overall quality of care.

One area where this integration is particularly impactful is in the management of dental caries. The traditional approach of carious tissue removal often involves extensive drilling and mechanical preparation, which, while effective in eradicating decay, can result in the loss of healthy tooth structure. Conversely, minimally invasive techniques such as air abrasion or laser therapy allow for targeted removal of carious tissue with less impact on the surrounding healthy enamel and dentin. Integrating these minimally invasive techniques with traditional restorative methods, such as composite resin fillings or crowns, offers a balanced approach that combines the precision of modern technology with the reliability of conventional methods. For example, a dentist might use laser therapy to remove decay from a tooth while preserving as much healthy structure as possible, and then apply a composite resin to restore the tooth, ensuring both effective treatment and minimal intervention.

The integration approach extends to the field of cosmetic dentistry as well. Traditional techniques for enhancing esthetics often involve significant alterations to tooth structure, such as the placement of crowns or veneers. However, with the advent of minimally invasive options like tooth whitening and direct composite bonding, clinicians can achieve significant esthetic improvements with less invasive procedures. Combining these methods allows for a more conservative approach to cosmetic enhancements. For instance, a patient seeking to improve the appearance of their smile might first undergo tooth whitening to address discoloration and then use direct composite bonding to correct minor imperfections. This sequential approach reduces the need for more extensive procedures and minimizes the impact on the natural tooth structure.

Another critical area where the integration of minimally invasive techniques with traditional methods proves beneficial is in the management of periodontal disease. Traditionally, periodontal therapy involved mechanical scaling and root planing to remove plaque and calculus from the tooth surfaces. While effective, this method can sometimes be invasive and uncomfortable for patients. The integration of laser therapy into periodontal treatment offers a less invasive alternative for decontaminating the periodontal tissues. By using lasers to target specific areas of infection, clinicians can complement traditional scaling and root planing, leading to improved outcomes and enhanced patient comfort. This combined approach not only addresses the microbial load but also promotes more effective healing of the periodontal tissues.

In the context of trauma management, integrating minimally invasive techniques with traditional methods allows for a comprehensive approach to treating dental injuries. For instance, in the case of a fractured tooth, a traditional approach might involve significant restorative work to repair the damage. However, minimally invasive techniques such as adhesive bonding can be employed to address smaller fractures or to stabilize the tooth before proceeding with more extensive restorations like crowns or onlays. This combination of methods ensures that the tooth is treated conservatively while still achieving the necessary repairs for function and esthetics.

The integration of these techniques also necessitates a nuanced understanding of the patient's individual needs and preferences. For example, some patients may have specific concerns about the invasiveness of certain procedures or may prefer to avoid more extensive treatments whenever possible. By integrating minimally invasive techniques with traditional methods, clinicians can offer tailored treatment plans that align with the patient's values and expectations. This patient-centered approach enhances satisfaction and compliance, leading to better overall outcomes.

Furthermore, effective integration requires ongoing education and training for dental professionals. Staying current with advancements in both minimally invasive and traditional techniques is crucial for ensuring that practitioners can apply the most appropriate methods for each clinical situation. Continuing education programs, hands-on workshops, and professional development opportunities are essential for mastering the integration of these techniques and for maintaining the highest standards of care.

In summary, the integration of minimally invasive techniques with traditional methods represents a sophisticated approach to dental care that leverages the strengths of both to optimize patient outcomes. By combining the precision and conservatism of minimally invasive techniques with the proven efficacy of traditional methods, clinicians can provide comprehensive, effective, and patient-centered care. This approach not only enhances clinical results but also aligns with the evolving standards of dental practice, ensuring that patients receive the best possible treatment while preserving the health and integrity of their natural teeth.

CHAPTER 25: PATIENT-CENTERED CARE AND COMMUNICATION IN MINIMALLY INVASIVE DENTISTRY

In the realm of minimally invasive dentistry, patient-centered care and effective communication are paramount for achieving optimal outcomes and ensuring a positive treatment experience. This chapter delves into how these principles apply to minimally invasive techniques, emphasizing the strategies that dental professionals can employ to engage patients, address their concerns, and enhance their understanding of treatment options.

Patient-centered care in minimally invasive dentistry revolves around a tailored approach that respects and responds to the individual needs and preferences of patients. This approach requires a deep understanding of the patient's values, concerns, and expectations, particularly when considering the benefits and limitations of minimally invasive techniques. A core aspect of patient-centered care is involving patients in their treatment decisions, which is facilitated by clear, transparent communication.

Effective communication begins with the initial patient consultation, where establishing a rapport and building trust is crucial. Dentists must listen actively to patients' concerns and questions about their dental health and treatment options. This dialogue should be open and non-judgmental, allowing patients to express their fears and preferences without reservation. By understanding the patient's perspective, clinicians can better align their treatment recommendations with the patient's values and goals.

Once a mutual understanding is established, it is essential to discuss the specific advantages of minimally invasive techniques. These techniques often offer benefits such as reduced discomfort, quicker recovery times, and the preservation of natural tooth structure. However, it is equally important to address any limitations or potential risks associated with these methods. Patients should be informed about the realistic outcomes and any potential need for follow-up treatments. Clear, honest communication helps set appropriate expectations and fosters a collaborative relationship between the patient and the clinician.

Another critical component of patient-centered care is patient education. Educating patients about the minimally invasive procedures, including how they work and what to expect, empowers them to make informed decisions about their dental care. Visual aids, such as diagrams or digital simulations, can be particularly useful in explaining complex procedures. Providing written information or access to reliable online resources can further support patient understanding and reinforce verbal explanations.

Moreover, discussing the preventive aspect of minimally invasive dentistry is vital. Patients should understand how preventive measures, such as regular check-ups, fluoride treatments, and sealants, contribute to long-term dental health and reduce the need for more invasive treatments. Emphasizing the proactive nature of these techniques helps patients appreciate their role in maintaining their oral health and encourages adherence to recommended preventive care.

Engaging patients in their treatment decisions involves not only providing information but also soliciting their input and preferences. Shared decision-making is a process where the clinician and patient collaborate to choose the best course of action, considering both medical evidence and the patient's personal values. This approach respects the patient's autonomy and promotes a sense of ownership over their dental care. When patients are actively involved in their treatment planning, they are more likely to be satisfied with their care and adhere to treatment recommendations.

Addressing patient concerns effectively also plays a significant role in patient-centered care. Minimally invasive techniques, while generally less traumatic, may still evoke anxiety or apprehension in some patients. Clinicians should be prepared to offer reassurance and answer any questions that arise. Techniques such as sedation or pain management options should be discussed openly if there are concerns about discomfort or anxiety. By acknowledging and addressing these concerns, clinicians can enhance patient comfort and trust.

In addition to verbal communication, non-verbal cues also influence the patient experience. A calm, empathetic demeanor, and a supportive environment contribute to a positive interaction. Clinicians should be attentive to the patient's body language and verbal feedback, adjusting their approach as needed to ensure the patient feels comfortable and heard.

Finally, follow-up care and communication are integral to maintaining a patient-centered approach. After a minimally invasive procedure, patients should be provided with clear instructions for post-treatment care and encouraged to reach out with any questions or concerns. Regular follow-up appointments allow for the monitoring of treatment outcomes and provide an opportunity for ongoing patient engagement. By maintaining open lines of communication, clinicians can address any issues that arise promptly and ensure continued patient satisfaction.

In summary, patient-centered care and effective communication are foundational elements in minimally invasive dentistry. By engaging patients in their treatment decisions, addressing their concerns, and ensuring they understand the benefits and limitations of minimally invasive techniques, dental professionals can enhance the overall patient experience and achieve better treatment outcomes. This approach not only fosters trust and satisfaction but also supports the successful implementation of minimally invasive techniques in achieving long-term oral health and well-being.

In the realm of minimally invasive dentistry, patient-centered care is integral to fostering positive outcomes and ensuring effective treatment. This approach not only focuses on the technical aspects of dental care but also emphasizes the importance of understanding and addressing the unique needs and preferences of each patient. Effective communication is a cornerstone of this approach, playing a pivotal role in the patient's overall experience and treatment success.

The essence of patient-centered care lies in the ability to tailor dental treatments to individual patients. This personalization involves recognizing each patient's specific concerns, health history, and treatment goals. By engaging in open dialogue, dental professionals can gain insights into the patient's expectations and anxieties, which are essential for creating a treatment plan that aligns with their values and preferences.

This dialogue also helps in building a trusting relationship between the patient and the clinician, which is crucial for successful outcomes.

One of the key strategies for engaging patients in their treatment decisions is providing clear and comprehensive information about the available options. In minimally invasive dentistry, where the emphasis is on preserving natural tooth structure and reducing intervention, patients need to understand how these techniques differ from traditional methods. Explaining the principles and advantages of minimally invasive approaches—such as less discomfort, shorter recovery times, and reduced need for extensive procedures—can help patients appreciate the value of these treatments. Additionally, presenting potential limitations or risks associated with these methods ensures that patients are fully informed and can make decisions based on a balanced understanding of their choices.

Effective communication also involves using language that is accessible and free of jargon. Medical terminology can be daunting or confusing for patients, so it is important to use simple, everyday language when discussing procedures and outcomes. Visual aids, such as diagrams, models, or digital simulations, can further enhance understanding by providing a tangible representation of the procedures being discussed. These tools can help demystify complex concepts and facilitate more informed decision-making.

Addressing patient concerns is another crucial aspect of patient-centered care. In minimally invasive dentistry, patients might have specific concerns related to the perceived effectiveness of new techniques, potential discomfort during procedures, or the long-term outcomes of their treatment. It is essential for clinicians to actively listen to these concerns, validate the patient's feelings, and provide thoughtful responses. For instance, if a patient is worried about the effectiveness of a minimally invasive treatment compared to more traditional methods, the clinician should provide evidence-based information and discuss how recent advancements have enhanced the efficacy of these approaches.

Moreover, managing patient anxiety and fear is vital for a positive treatment experience. Dental anxiety can significantly impact a patient's willingness to undergo necessary procedures and can affect their overall treatment outcome. Clinicians should be prepared to offer reassurance and discuss strategies for managing anxiety, such as sedation options or relaxation techniques. Acknowledging and addressing these emotional aspects can help in creating a more comfortable and trusting environment for the patient.

Patient education extends beyond the initial consultation and involves ongoing communication throughout the treatment process. After a minimally invasive procedure, providing clear post-treatment care instructions and being available to answer any follow-up questions is essential. Patients should be informed about what to expect during their recovery, any signs of complications to watch for, and the importance of adhering to prescribed care routines. Regular follow-up appointments offer an opportunity to monitor progress, address any concerns that may arise, and reinforce the importance of continuing with preventive care.

Engaging patients in their care also means respecting their autonomy and preferences. Shared decision-making is a collaborative process where the clinician and patient work together to determine the most appropriate treatment plan. This approach ensures that patients feel valued and empowered in their healthcare decisions, leading to higher satisfaction and better adherence to treatment plans. It is important to consider the patient's lifestyle, personal preferences, and treatment goals when developing a care plan.

Finally, the integration of patient feedback is an essential component of patient-centered care. Collecting and analyzing patient feedback on their experience with minimally invasive procedures can provide valuable insights into areas for improvement. Feedback mechanisms, such as surveys or direct communication, allow dental practices to make informed adjustments to their approach, enhance patient satisfaction, and continuously improve the quality of care.

In conclusion, patient-centered care and effective communication are foundational to the practice of minimally invasive dentistry. By engaging patients in their treatment decisions, addressing their concerns, and ensuring that they understand the benefits and limitations of minimally invasive approaches, dental professionals can enhance the patient experience and achieve better treatment outcomes. This holistic approach not only supports the technical aspects of care but also fosters a supportive, empathetic relationship between the clinician and patient, ultimately leading to a more successful and satisfying dental care experience.

Incorporating patient-centered care and effective communication into minimally invasive dentistry requires a nuanced understanding of patient dynamics and an ability to tailor interactions to individual needs. This approach is not merely a matter of enhancing patient satisfaction but is integral to achieving optimal clinical outcomes. By focusing on the patient's perspective and actively involving them in their care, dental professionals can create a more collaborative and supportive treatment environment.

The process of engaging patients in their treatment decisions begins with establishing a strong rapport and understanding their unique concerns and preferences. It is essential for dental professionals to create an open and inviting atmosphere where patients feel comfortable expressing their thoughts and asking questions. This can be facilitated by adopting a conversational approach rather than a purely clinical one, ensuring that the patient's voice is heard and considered throughout the treatment process.

When discussing treatment options, particularly in the context of minimally invasive dentistry, clarity is key. Patients must be provided with comprehensive information about the available treatments, including how each option aligns with their specific needs and circumstances. For instance, when presenting the benefits of a minimally invasive approach compared to more traditional methods, it is important to highlight not only the technical advantages but also how these benefits translate into real-world outcomes, such as reduced recovery time and improved long-term health.

In addition to explaining the benefits, it is crucial to address any limitations or potential risks associated with minimally invasive techniques. Transparency in discussing the potential downsides of any treatment option helps in setting realistic expectations and fosters trust between the patient and clinician. This balanced approach ensures that patients are well-informed and can make decisions that align with their personal health goals and comfort levels.

A key aspect of patient-centered care is ensuring that patients fully understand their treatment options and the implications of their choices. This involves breaking down complex information into understandable segments and using visual aids, such as diagrams or digital simulations, to illustrate procedures. Such tools can enhance comprehension and help patients visualize the outcomes of different treatment options, which is particularly useful in minimally invasive dentistry where techniques and technologies can be intricate and unfamiliar.

Active listening is another essential component of effective communication. Dental professionals should be attentive to patient concerns, demonstrating empathy and understanding. This involves not only hearing what patients say but also interpreting their non-verbal cues and emotional responses. For example, if a patient expresses anxiety about a particular procedure, acknowledging their fears and providing reassurance can significantly impact their comfort level and willingness to proceed with the treatment.

In managing patient expectations, it is important to provide realistic projections of treatment outcomes. While minimally invasive techniques are designed to be less disruptive and more conservative, patients should be made aware that results can vary based on individual factors, such as the extent of dental issues and overall oral health. By setting realistic expectations and discussing potential variations in outcomes, dental professionals can help patients make informed decisions and reduce the likelihood of dissatisfaction.

Patient education extends beyond the initial consultation and includes ongoing communication throughout the treatment and recovery phases. After a minimally invasive procedure, clear instructions for post-treatment care are vital. Patients should be informed about what to expect during recovery, any necessary follow-up appointments, and signs of complications to watch for. Providing written materials or digital resources can complement verbal instructions and serve as a reference for patients as they navigate their recovery.

Moreover, incorporating feedback mechanisms into the practice can further enhance patient-centered care. Soliciting feedback from patients about their experience with minimally invasive procedures allows dental professionals to identify areas for improvement and address any issues that may arise. This feedback loop not only helps in refining practice protocols but also demonstrates a commitment to patient satisfaction and continuous improvement.

In conclusion, patient-centered care and effective communication are integral to the success of minimally invasive dentistry. By engaging patients in their treatment decisions, addressing their concerns with empathy and clarity, and ensuring they understand the benefits and limitations of various approaches, dental professionals can enhance the overall patient experience. This collaborative approach not only supports the technical aspects of care but also fosters a trusting and supportive relationship between the clinician and patient, ultimately leading to better outcomes and higher levels of patient satisfaction.

CHAPTER 26: MANAGING COMPLICATIONS IN MINIMALLY INVASIVE DENTISTRY

In minimally invasive dentistry, the focus on conservative approaches often leads to favorable outcomes and enhanced patient experiences. However, even with the best techniques and precautions, complications can arise, necessitating a thorough understanding of how to manage and mitigate these issues. Effective management of complications not only preserves the integrity of minimally invasive treatments but also ensures optimal patient outcomes and maintains trust in conservative approaches.

One common complication that may occur in minimally invasive dentistry is the failure of adhesive or restorative materials. These materials, which are integral to many minimally invasive procedures such as bonding and composite restorations, can occasionally fail to adhere properly or exhibit premature degradation. Such failures may be attributed to factors such as improper application, contamination, or inadequate curing. To manage these issues, it is essential to first identify the root cause of the failure. Rigorous attention to detail during the preparation and application phases can prevent such complications. For instance, ensuring that the tooth surface is thoroughly cleaned and dried before applying adhesive can significantly enhance the bond strength. Additionally, using light-curing units with appropriate intensity and wavelength is crucial for optimal material polymerization.

Another potential issue is sensitivity following minimally invasive procedures, particularly those involving the removal of decayed tissue or preparation of the tooth structure. Sensitivity can arise due to the exposure of dentinal tubules or the application of restorative materials that are not fully compatible with the tooth structure. To manage post-operative sensitivity, practitioners can employ desensitizing agents or varnishes that occlude dentinal tubules and reduce nerve exposure. Moreover, advising patients on proper oral hygiene practices and the use of desensitizing toothpaste can help alleviate sensitivity over time.

Complications can also arise from procedural errors or unforeseen patient reactions. For example, during the placement of veneers or direct restorations, complications such as improper fit or color mismatch may occur. These issues can be managed by conducting thorough pre-procedural planning and using diagnostic tools such as digital imaging and mock-ups to visualize the outcome before actual placement. In cases where complications do arise, adjustments or remakes of the restorations may be necessary to achieve the desired esthetic and functional results.

In the realm of minimally invasive periodontal procedures, complications may include issues such as infection or inadequate tissue response. For instance, in procedures such as laser-assisted gingival contouring or subgingival debridement, complications may involve the development of localized infections or delayed healing. Effective management involves implementing strict infection control measures, such as using sterile instruments and maintaining a clean clinical environment. Post-operative care instructions should be clear and comprehensive, including guidelines on oral hygiene and the use of antimicrobial agents if necessary.

Moreover, it is important to recognize and address patient-specific factors that may contribute to complications. For instance, patients with compromised immune systems or those who are not compliant with oral hygiene recommendations may be at higher risk for complications following minimally invasive procedures. Tailoring treatment plans to accommodate these factors and providing additional support and monitoring can help mitigate potential issues.

Complications associated with minimally invasive procedures can also include issues related to patient discomfort or anxiety. Although minimally invasive techniques are designed to be less invasive and more comfortable, some patients may still experience discomfort during or after the procedure. Addressing these concerns involves providing adequate pain management options, such as local anesthesia or analgesics, and offering reassurance and support throughout the treatment process. Clear communication about what to expect and providing follow-up care can help alleviate patient anxiety and enhance the overall treatment experience.

Prevention is a crucial aspect of managing complications. Implementing best practices in clinical techniques, using high-quality materials, and adhering to standardized protocols can significantly reduce the likelihood of complications. Continuous professional development and staying abreast of advances in minimally invasive techniques also contribute to effective complication management. Regular review of clinical cases, including any complications encountered, can provide valuable insights and contribute to improved practice and patient outcomes.

In summary, managing complications in minimally invasive dentistry requires a comprehensive approach that includes understanding potential issues, implementing preventive measures, and applying effective management strategies when problems arise. By addressing complications promptly and effectively, dental practitioners can uphold the principles of minimally invasive dentistry while ensuring high-quality patient care and maintaining confidence in conservative treatment approaches.

In minimally invasive dentistry, effective management of complications requires a proactive and methodical approach. The complexity of dental procedures, even when minimally invasive, often presents unique challenges that necessitate a nuanced understanding of both the techniques and their potential pitfalls. Addressing complications involves not only reactive measures but also a preventive mindset to minimize the risk of adverse outcomes.

One significant aspect of complication management involves the careful monitoring of patient responses to minimally invasive treatments. For instance, patients who undergo procedures such as air abrasion or laser treatments may experience variations in their reactions based on individual sensitivity and healing responses. Post-procedural discomfort or reactions can be mitigated by establishing clear protocols for patient evaluation and follow-up. Regular post-treatment assessments enable the early detection of any emerging issues, allowing for timely intervention and adjustment of treatment plans as needed. This approach not only addresses complications as they arise but also contributes to the refinement of techniques based on patient feedback and outcomes.

Another area of concern is the management of complications related to material interactions. Minimally invasive techniques often involve the use of advanced materials, such as composites, adhesives, or biomimetic substances, which can interact with the natural tooth structure in complex ways. For instance, the failure of a composite restoration may occur due to inadequate bonding, leading to issues such as marginal leakage or secondary caries. Effective management requires a thorough understanding of material properties and their interactions with tooth substrates. Rigorous adherence to application protocols, including proper surface preparation and curing techniques, can reduce the likelihood of material-related complications. Additionally, selecting materials that are well-matched to the clinical situation and patient needs enhances the long-term success of the treatment.

Complications in minimally invasive procedures may also involve issues related to the accuracy and precision of techniques. For example, when performing conservative cavity preparations or direct restorations, achieving optimal contours and margins is crucial for both functional and esthetic outcomes. Inaccuracies in these areas can result in problems such as plaque accumulation or compromised function. Employing advanced diagnostic tools, such as digital imaging or intraoral scanners, can improve the precision of minimally invasive procedures and reduce the incidence of related complications. Additionally, incorporating techniques such as magnification and enhanced lighting into clinical practice can further refine the accuracy of procedures and minimize the risk of errors.

Patient-specific factors are another critical element in managing complications. Variations in individual anatomy, systemic health conditions, and behavioral factors can influence treatment outcomes. For instance, patients with dental anxiety or those who are non-compliant with oral hygiene practices may experience higher rates of complications. Addressing these factors involves a personalized approach to patient care, including detailed assessments and tailored treatment plans. Educating patients about the importance of post-procedural care, providing clear instructions, and offering support for managing anxiety or other concerns can significantly impact the success of minimally invasive treatments.

Effective communication between the dental team and patients plays a pivotal role in complication management. Transparent discussions about potential risks and expected outcomes of minimally invasive procedures help set realistic expectations and foster patient trust. Ensuring that patients are well-informed about the steps involved in their treatment, as well as any necessary follow-up care, empowers them to participate actively in their own recovery and management. This collaborative approach not only enhances patient satisfaction but also contributes to better overall treatment outcomes.

In cases where complications do arise, a systematic approach to their management is essential. This involves identifying the underlying causes, implementing corrective measures, and closely monitoring the patient's progress. For instance, if a minimally invasive procedure leads to persistent discomfort or adverse reactions, a detailed investigation into potential contributing factors, such as technique errors or material issues, should be conducted. Based on the findings, appropriate adjustments to the treatment plan can be made, including the use of alternative materials or modified techniques. Prompt and effective resolution of complications helps to restore patient comfort and maintain the integrity of the minimally invasive approach.

Furthermore, continuous education and professional development are vital for managing complications effectively. Staying updated with the latest advancements in minimally invasive techniques and materials allows practitioners to incorporate new knowledge and strategies into their practice. Participating in training sessions, workshops, and peer-reviewed research enhances one's ability to anticipate and address potential complications, ultimately leading to improved patient care and clinical outcomes.

In summary, managing complications in minimally invasive dentistry involves a comprehensive and proactive approach that addresses both preventive and reactive aspects of care. By closely monitoring patient responses, understanding material interactions, ensuring procedural accuracy, and considering patient-specific factors, dental practitioners can effectively manage and mitigate complications. Clear communication, systematic problem-solving, and ongoing professional development further contribute to the successful integration of minimally invasive techniques, ensuring that they continue to offer safe and effective solutions for a wide range of dental conditions.

In the realm of minimally invasive dentistry, managing complications effectively is crucial for maintaining patient trust and ensuring the success of dental interventions. As these techniques become more sophisticated, understanding and addressing potential complications is key to optimizing patient outcomes and preserving the benefits of a minimally invasive approach.

A fundamental aspect of managing complications is the early recognition of issues that may arise from minimally invasive procedures. Despite the conservative nature of these techniques, challenges such as sensitivity, treatment failure, or discomfort can still occur. Early detection through regular follow-up appointments and vigilant patient monitoring is essential. This includes assessing the initial response to treatment, evaluating any signs of complications, and promptly addressing any concerns raised by the patient. For instance, if a patient reports increased sensitivity following a procedure, it is important to differentiate whether this is a normal part of the healing process or indicative of an underlying problem such as improper bonding or residual caries. A thorough examination and diagnostic evaluation can help determine the appropriate course of action.

Treatment failures, although rare with minimally invasive techniques, can still occur due to factors such as inadequate material application or misalignment. For example, the failure of a minimally invasive composite restoration might be attributed to improper curing, leading to issues such as early wear or debonding. To mitigate such risks, adherence to manufacturer guidelines and established protocols is critical. This includes ensuring that all materials are applied under optimal conditions, such as appropriate light curing times and environmental factors. Additionally, employing techniques such as magnification and enhanced visualization can help in achieving precise material application and preventing errors.

In some cases, adverse reactions may arise due to patient-specific factors or interactions between the dental materials and the tooth structure. For example, allergic reactions to dental materials, though uncommon, can cause significant discomfort and necessitate immediate attention. Addressing such reactions involves identifying the offending material, providing symptomatic relief, and selecting alternative materials that are compatible with the patient's sensitivity profile. Comprehensive patient histories, including any known allergies or sensitivities, should be reviewed prior to initiating treatment to minimize the risk of such reactions.

In managing complications related to the long-term durability of minimally invasive treatments, it is important to consider both the technical and biological aspects. The longevity of materials such as composites and adhesives can be influenced by factors such as oral hygiene, dietary habits, and occlusal forces. Educating patients about the importance of maintaining good oral hygiene, avoiding excessive consumption of staining agents or hard foods, and scheduling regular dental check-ups can significantly impact the success and longevity of minimally invasive restorations. Regular monitoring and maintenance of restorations are also vital for identifying and addressing issues such as wear or marginal leakage before they lead to more significant complications.

Another critical component of complication management is the use of evidence-based protocols and continuous professional development. Staying informed about the latest advancements in minimally invasive techniques and materials helps practitioners apply the most current and effective methods. Engaging in continuing education, attending professional workshops, and reviewing the latest research findings contribute to an enhanced understanding of potential complications and their management. This ongoing learning process enables practitioners to refine their techniques and adapt to new challenges effectively.

In addition to technical and procedural considerations, the role of patient communication cannot be overstated. Transparent and open communication with patients about the potential risks and expected outcomes of minimally invasive procedures fosters a collaborative relationship and enhances patient satisfaction. Providing detailed explanations of the procedure, potential complications, and post-treatment care instructions helps manage patient expectations and encourages proactive involvement in their own care. Addressing patient concerns promptly and empathetically further strengthens trust and compliance, contributing to better overall treatment outcomes.

In cases where complications are complex or persist despite initial management efforts, referral to a specialist or interdisciplinary team may be necessary. For example, cases involving severe or unusual reactions might benefit from the expertise of an allergist or a specialist in restorative dentistry. Collaboration with other healthcare providers ensures that all aspects of the patient's condition are addressed comprehensively, enhancing the likelihood of successful resolution.

In summary, the effective management of complications in minimally invasive dentistry involves a multifaceted approach that combines early detection, adherence to best practices, patient education, and ongoing professional development. By staying vigilant and responsive to potential issues, practitioners can maintain the integrity of minimally invasive techniques and ensure optimal outcomes for their patients. The integration of evidence-based strategies and clear communication further supports the successful application of minimally invasive dentistry, preserving its benefits while addressing any challenges that may arise.

CHAPTER 27: THE ROLE OF PREVENTIVE MEASURES IN MINIMALLY INVASIVE DENTISTRY

Preventive measures are fundamental to the philosophy of minimally invasive dentistry, emphasizing the reduction of dental issues before they necessitate more invasive interventions. By focusing on prevention, dental professionals can enhance patient outcomes, minimize the need for extensive treatments, and support the overarching goals of minimally invasive approaches. This chapter delves into how preventive protocols, patient education, and lifestyle modifications play a crucial role in maintaining oral health and aligning with minimally invasive principles.

The cornerstone of preventive care in minimally invasive dentistry is the implementation of comprehensive preventive protocols. These protocols are designed to proactively address common dental problems such as caries, periodontal disease, and enamel erosion, thus minimizing the need for restorative procedures. A proactive approach involves regular dental check-ups, which enable early detection of potential issues. Routine examinations and cleanings help identify early signs of decay or gum disease, allowing for timely intervention with conservative measures such as fluoride treatments or sealants. The use of diagnostic tools such as digital radiography and intraoral cameras further enhances the ability to detect problems before they escalate, facilitating early and less invasive treatments.

Patient education is equally pivotal in the preventive paradigm of minimally invasive dentistry. Educating patients about oral hygiene practices, dietary choices, and the impact of lifestyle habits is essential for empowering them to take an active role in their dental health. Effective communication strategies include explaining the significance of daily brushing and flossing, the benefits of using fluoride toothpaste, and the importance of regular dental visits. Additionally, providing information on how to manage dietary habits—such as reducing sugar intake and avoiding acidic foods—can significantly influence the development of dental issues. Engaging patients in their own care through personalized advice and demonstrations can lead to improved adherence to preventive practices and a greater understanding of the rationale behind them.

Lifestyle modifications are an integral component of preventive measures in minimally invasive dentistry. Lifestyle factors such as smoking, excessive alcohol consumption, and poor dietary choices can adversely affect oral health and increase the risk of dental problems. Addressing these factors through targeted interventions can help mitigate their impact. For example, offering resources and support for smoking cessation can contribute to better periodontal health and reduce the likelihood of oral cancer. Similarly, advising patients on the risks associated with excessive alcohol consumption and providing strategies for moderation can enhance overall oral health. By incorporating lifestyle counseling into patient care, dental professionals can support patients in making choices that benefit their long-term oral health.

Preventive measures also encompass the use of advanced technologies and treatments designed to enhance oral health and prevent the need for invasive procedures. For instance, the application of fluoride varnishes and dental sealants has been shown to significantly reduce the incidence of caries, particularly in high-risk populations. These treatments act as barriers to decay, protecting vulnerable tooth surfaces and reducing the likelihood of future restorative needs. Additionally, the use of minimally invasive diagnostic technologies such as laser fluorescence and digital caries detection systems allows for more accurate assessment of tooth health, enabling targeted preventive measures.

Integrating preventive strategies into daily practice requires a systematic approach that involves both the dental team and the patient. Establishing a routine for preventive care that includes regular screenings, professional cleanings, and tailored advice can help maintain oral health and prevent the progression of dental issues. Utilizing electronic health records to track patient history and treatment outcomes also supports a more effective preventive strategy by enabling the identification of patterns and trends that may indicate the need for additional preventive measures.

Collaboration between dental professionals and other healthcare providers can further enhance the effectiveness of preventive care. For example, working with pediatricians to promote oral health in children and collaborating with nutritionists to address dietary factors can create a more comprehensive approach to prevention. By extending preventive efforts beyond the dental office and incorporating interdisciplinary strategies, the overall impact on patient health can be significantly improved.

In conclusion, preventive measures are integral to the success of minimally invasive dentistry, offering a proactive approach to maintaining oral health and reducing the need for invasive treatments. Through the implementation of preventive protocols, patient education, and lifestyle modifications, dental professionals can significantly impact patient outcomes and support the goals of minimally invasive practices. Emphasizing prevention not only enhances the effectiveness of dental care but also aligns with the fundamental principles of minimally invasive dentistry, ultimately contributing to better oral health and improved quality of life for patients.

A significant aspect of preventive measures in minimally invasive dentistry is the emphasis on the early detection and management of dental conditions before they necessitate invasive treatments. Early diagnosis plays a crucial role in preventing the escalation of dental issues. Utilizing advanced diagnostic tools allows for a more precise and less invasive approach to identifying potential problems. For instance, digital radiography and advanced imaging technologies can reveal early signs of dental caries or periodontal disease that may not be visible during a routine clinical examination. These technologies provide high-resolution images with minimal radiation exposure, facilitating early intervention and reducing the need for more extensive treatments later on.

The integration of risk assessment tools into preventive care further enhances the effectiveness of minimally invasive practices. Risk assessment involves evaluating a patient's individual risk factors for developing dental issues, such as caries or gum disease. By identifying these risk factors, dental professionals can tailor preventive strategies to the specific needs of each patient. For example, patients with a high risk of caries might benefit from more frequent fluoride treatments or sealant applications, while those at risk for periodontal disease may require more intensive periodontal cleanings and patient education on proper oral hygiene techniques.

Preventive care also involves the use of caries management by risk assessment (CAMBRA) protocols, which focus on understanding and mitigating the risk factors that contribute to dental caries. CAMBRA protocols include evaluating factors such as oral hygiene practices, dietary habits, and socioeconomic status. By addressing these factors through targeted preventive measures, dental professionals can effectively reduce the incidence of carious lesions and support long-term oral health. This approach aligns with the principles of minimally invasive dentistry by focusing on preserving tooth structure and preventing the need for restorative interventions.

Patient involvement in preventive care is another critical component. Engaging patients in their own oral health management helps reinforce the importance of preventive practices and encourages adherence to recommended protocols. Involving patients in discussions about their oral health and treatment options fosters a collaborative relationship between the dental team and the patient. This collaborative approach can lead to better adherence to preventive measures and more successful outcomes.

Behavioral modifications are often necessary to achieve optimal preventive results. Behavioral interventions might include strategies for improving oral hygiene routines, dietary changes, or smoking cessation. For example, patients who consume high levels of sugary foods and beverages may need guidance on reducing their sugar intake and making healthier dietary choices. Similarly, patients who smoke or use tobacco products may benefit from targeted counseling and support to quit. Addressing these behavioral factors not only contributes to better oral health but also enhances the overall effectiveness of preventive measures.

The role of fluoride in preventive dentistry cannot be overstated. Fluoride treatments, including topical applications and fluoride toothpaste, help strengthen tooth enamel and make it more resistant to acid attacks. Regular fluoride treatments are particularly beneficial for patients at high risk for caries, such as those with a history of frequent cavities or those with limited access to dental care. Fluoride varnishes and gels are commonly used in both pediatric and adult patients to provide additional protection against carious lesions.

Sealants represent another effective preventive measure, especially for pediatric patients. Dental sealants are thin, protective coatings applied to the chewing surfaces of molars and premolars. These sealants act as a barrier, preventing plaque and food particles from accumulating in the deep grooves and fissures of the teeth. By sealing these areas, dental professionals can significantly reduce the risk of caries development, especially in children who may be more susceptible to cavities.

Incorporating preventive care into the overall treatment plan requires a holistic approach that considers both the patient's individual needs and the latest advancements in dental technology. Developing and implementing preventive protocols should be a continuous process that evolves with emerging research and technological advancements. Dental professionals must stay informed about the latest evidence-based practices and integrate these into their preventive care strategies to ensure the highest level of patient care.

To maximize the benefits of preventive care, it is essential for dental practices to create an environment that supports and encourages preventive measures. This includes providing patients with clear information about the importance of preventive care, offering convenient access to preventive treatments, and fostering a positive and proactive approach to oral health. By creating a supportive environment and prioritizing preventive care, dental professionals can significantly impact patient outcomes and align with the goals of minimally invasive dentistry.

In summary, the role of preventive measures in minimally invasive dentistry is vital for reducing the need for invasive treatments and promoting long-term oral health. Through the implementation of comprehensive preventive protocols, patient education, and lifestyle modifications, dental professionals can effectively manage dental issues before they require more extensive interventions. By focusing on early detection, risk assessment, and patient involvement, preventive care supports the principles of minimally invasive dentistry and contributes to optimal patient outcomes.

The success of preventive measures in minimally invasive dentistry hinges on a multi-faceted approach that integrates scientific advancements, patient education, and consistent clinical practice. The integration of evidence-based preventive protocols into daily dental practice ensures that patients receive the most effective and current care available. This approach not only improves patient outcomes but also aligns with the overarching goals of minimally invasive dentistry, which emphasizes the preservation of natural tooth structure and the prevention of extensive interventions.

One of the cornerstones of preventive care is the regular application of fluoride. Fluoride's role in enhancing enamel resistance to demineralization and promoting remineralization of early carious lesions is well-documented. Professional fluoride treatments, such as fluoride varnishes and gels, offer a concentrated dose that can provide additional protection beyond what is available from over-the-counter products. This is particularly important for patients who are at a higher risk of caries due to factors such as poor oral hygiene, high sugar consumption, or specific medical conditions.

In addition to fluoride treatments, the use of dental sealants has proven to be an effective preventive measure, especially in pediatric patients. Sealants are applied to the occlusal surfaces of molars and premolars to fill and protect the deep grooves and pits where decay often starts. By creating a barrier that prevents plaque accumulation and food particles from settling into these vulnerable areas, sealants play a crucial role in reducing the incidence of carious lesions in young patients.

Beyond these specific interventions, a comprehensive preventive strategy must include patient education and lifestyle modification. Educating patients about the importance of daily oral hygiene practices—such as brushing twice daily with fluoride toothpaste, flossing, and using mouth rinses—empowers them to take an active role in maintaining their oral health. Clear communication about the consequences of neglecting these practices and the benefits of adherence is essential in fostering patient compliance.

Lifestyle modifications also play a significant role in preventive dentistry. For example, dietary counseling to reduce the intake of sugary and acidic foods can significantly impact oral health. Sugars and acids are primary contributors to tooth decay and erosion, and modifying dietary habits can help mitigate these risks. Additionally, smoking cessation programs are crucial for patients who use tobacco products, as smoking is a known risk factor for periodontal disease and oral cancer.

The use of caries risk assessment tools further enhances the effectiveness of preventive strategies. These tools help clinicians evaluate a patient's likelihood of developing carious lesions based on various factors, such as their oral hygiene practices, dietary habits, and previous dental history. By assessing these risk factors, dental professionals can tailor preventive measures to address the specific needs of each patient, thus optimizing their oral health outcomes.

Regular dental check-ups and professional cleanings are integral to preventive care. During these visits, dental professionals can monitor for early signs of dental issues and provide timely interventions. Professional cleanings help remove plaque and tartar that patients may not be able to eliminate through brushing and flossing alone. These appointments also offer an opportunity for dental professionals to reinforce preventive strategies and make any necessary adjustments to the patient's care plan.

The integration of preventive care into minimally invasive dentistry also involves leveraging technological advancements. Digital imaging technologies, such as intraoral cameras and advanced radiographic systems, allow for the early detection of dental issues with minimal discomfort for patients. These technologies facilitate the diagnosis of problems at their earliest stages, enabling prompt and less invasive treatment options.

Furthermore, the development of new materials and techniques continues to advance the field of preventive dentistry. Innovations such as bioactive materials, which release fluoride or calcium to aid in remineralization, and novel adhesive systems that improve the longevity of sealants, contribute to more effective preventive care. Staying abreast of these advancements ensures that dental practices can provide the highest standard of care and integrate the latest preventive measures into their practice.

Overall, the role of preventive measures in minimally invasive dentistry is critical for reducing the need for more extensive treatments and promoting long-term oral health. By implementing evidence-based protocols, engaging patients in their oral health care, and continuously adapting to advancements in dental science, dental professionals can significantly enhance patient outcomes and align with the principles of minimally invasive dentistry. The focus on prevention not only improves the quality of care but also supports a proactive approach to maintaining oral health, ultimately benefiting both patients and dental practices.

CHAPTER 28: INNOVATIONS AND FUTURE DIRECTIONS IN MINIMALLY INVASIVE DENTISTRY

As minimally invasive dentistry continues to evolve, the future promises a wealth of innovations that are set to transform the landscape of dental practice. The integration of emerging technologies, the development of new materials, and the refinement of techniques are all poised to further enhance the efficacy and patient-centered focus of minimally invasive dentistry. This chapter explores these advancements and anticipates how they will shape the future of dental care.

One of the most exciting areas of innovation is the advancement of digital technologies. Digital imaging systems, including cone-beam computed tomography (CBCT) and digital intraoral cameras, are revolutionizing diagnostics and treatment planning. These technologies offer high-resolution images with reduced radiation exposure, enabling precise diagnosis and tailored treatment strategies. Future developments in imaging technology are expected to further enhance diagnostic capabilities, providing even more detailed and accurate assessments of dental structures.

Similarly, the incorporation of artificial intelligence (AI) in dentistry holds great promise. AI algorithms are increasingly being used to analyze large datasets of patient information, including radiographic images, to assist in diagnosis and treatment planning. These systems can identify patterns and anomalies that may be subtle or difficult for human eyes to detect, thereby enhancing diagnostic accuracy and early intervention. As AI technology continues to advance, it is likely to become an integral part of diagnostic and treatment workflows, offering valuable support to clinicians and improving patient outcomes.

Another significant advancement is the development of innovative biomaterials. New materials are being designed to enhance the durability and functionality of dental restorations while minimizing invasiveness. For instance, bioactive materials that promote natural remineralization and support the repair of damaged tissues are gaining traction. These materials not only improve the longevity of restorations but also contribute to the overall health of the tooth structure. Additionally, advancements in adhesive technologies are making it possible to achieve stronger and more reliable bonds between restorative materials and tooth enamel or dentin.

The field of regenerative dentistry is also advancing, with new techniques and materials that aim to restore lost dental structures and function. Stem cell research and tissue engineering are at the forefront of these developments, offering the potential for regenerative treatments that could one day replace damaged or lost teeth with biologically viable alternatives. These innovations could significantly reduce the need for traditional invasive procedures and offer more natural and effective solutions for dental restoration.

In parallel with these technological advancements, there is a growing emphasis on personalized care. Advances in genomics and patient-specific data are enabling more tailored approaches to dental treatment. By understanding an individual's genetic predispositions and specific risk factors, clinicians can customize preventive and therapeutic strategies to address each patient's unique needs. This personalized approach not only enhances the effectiveness of treatments but also supports a more patient-centered model of care.

The integration of telemedicine in dentistry is another noteworthy trend. Tele-dentistry platforms allow for remote consultations, follow-up appointments, and even real-time monitoring of certain conditions. This technology can increase access to dental care, particularly for patients in remote or underserved areas, and provide greater convenience for patients managing chronic conditions. As tele-dentistry continues to develop, it is likely to become a more prominent aspect of dental care delivery, complementing traditional in-person visits and expanding the reach of minimally invasive techniques.

Furthermore, advancements in laser technology are continuing to refine minimally invasive procedures. Lasers are increasingly used for various dental treatments, including soft tissue management, caries removal, and teeth whitening. Future innovations in laser technology are expected to enhance precision, reduce discomfort, and accelerate healing, further aligning with the principles of minimally invasive dentistry.

In terms of technique refinement, there is ongoing research into optimizing current minimally invasive methods and exploring new procedural approaches. For instance, advances in adhesive dentistry and minimally invasive endodontics are contributing to more effective and less invasive treatments. Techniques such as micro-invasive caries management and conservative root canal therapies are being continually improved to minimize the extent of intervention while maximizing therapeutic outcomes.

The future of minimally invasive dentistry is also likely to see increased integration of interdisciplinary approaches. Collaboration among dental specialists, including periodontists, orthodontists, and prosthodontists, can lead to more comprehensive and coordinated care. Such interdisciplinary strategies can enhance the application of minimally invasive techniques across various areas of dentistry, resulting in better patient outcomes and more cohesive treatment plans.

As these innovations unfold, the field of minimally invasive dentistry is set to become even more dynamic and patient-focused. Embracing new technologies, materials, and techniques will not only improve the precision and effectiveness of dental treatments but also ensure that care remains aligned with the principles of minimal intervention and optimal patient outcomes. The continued evolution of minimally invasive dentistry reflects a commitment to advancing the field and enhancing the quality of care provided to patients.

The exploration of future innovations in minimally invasive dentistry reveals a field poised for transformative advancements. As technology continues to evolve, new methodologies and materials will likely redefine how dental care is delivered, further advancing the core principles of minimally invasive dentistry.

Among the forefront of these innovations is the development of advanced diagnostic tools. Enhanced imaging technologies, including more refined versions of cone-beam computed tomography (CBCT) and optical coherence tomography (OCT), promise even greater precision in diagnosing dental conditions. These tools offer detailed three-dimensional views of dental structures, allowing for more accurate assessment and early detection of issues. Future iterations are expected to integrate with AI-driven analysis, providing real-time diagnostic support and predictive analytics to anticipate dental issues before they develop into more significant problems.

Another promising area is the refinement of minimally invasive restorative materials. Advances in material science are leading to the creation of novel biomaterials with superior properties. For instance, next-generation composite resins are being developed with enhanced aesthetic qualities, improved wear resistance, and greater compatibility with tooth structure. These materials are designed to provide longer-lasting and more natural-looking restorations while adhering to minimally invasive principles. Additionally, the development of smart materials that can actively respond to environmental changes, such as pH variations or stress, is on the horizon, potentially offering adaptive solutions to varying clinical scenarios.

The use of regenerative techniques is also advancing rapidly. Stem cell research and tissue engineering are paving the way for innovative approaches to dental repair and regeneration. The application of stem cell therapy could eventually allow for the regeneration of lost or damaged dental tissues, including dentin and pulp, reducing the need for more invasive procedures. This could also extend to the development of biologically engineered dental implants that more closely mimic natural tooth structure and function.

Moreover, advancements in laser technology are expected to further enhance minimally invasive treatments. Lasers are already used in a variety of dental procedures for their precision and ability to minimize tissue damage. Emerging laser technologies promise even finer control and the ability to perform more complex procedures with minimal discomfort and quicker healing times. These advancements are likely to expand the range of conditions that can be effectively managed with laser technology, reinforcing the minimally invasive approach.

Digital workflows and the integration of virtual reality (VR) and augmented reality (AR) into dental practice represent another exciting frontier. VR and AR can be used for both patient education and surgical planning. For instance, AR can overlay digital images onto a patient's oral structures during treatment, aiding in real-time decision-making and increasing the accuracy of interventions. Similarly, VR can be employed to simulate complex procedures, providing clinicians with hands-on training and improving their skill sets without patient risk.

Tele-dentistry is also anticipated to evolve significantly. As remote consultation and monitoring technologies improve, they will offer expanded opportunities for managing dental health outside of traditional office settings. Future tele-dentistry platforms may include more sophisticated remote diagnostic tools, enabling real-time monitoring of oral health conditions and facilitating proactive management of potential issues. This could enhance access to care, particularly for patients in remote or underserved areas, and support ongoing patient engagement and education.

The convergence of artificial intelligence with digital dentistry continues to show great potential. AI-driven diagnostic tools and treatment planning systems are becoming more sophisticated, capable of analyzing vast amounts of data to provide personalized treatment recommendations. These systems can integrate patient history, current clinical findings, and predictive analytics to optimize treatment plans. As AI technology advances, it is likely to become increasingly integral to clinical decision-making, offering valuable insights and improving overall treatment outcomes.

Finally, the growing emphasis on patient-centered care

will drive the development of more customized and patient-specific approaches in minimally invasive dentistry. Innovations in personalized dental care will likely involve tailored preventive measures, individualized treatment plans, and enhanced patient engagement strategies. This shift towards personalized care will be supported by advancements in data collection and analysis, enabling more precise and effective management of each patient's unique oral health needs.

In conclusion, the future of minimally invasive dentistry is marked by a series of promising innovations that aim to refine and expand the scope of dental care. With advancements in diagnostic technology, materials science, regenerative techniques, and digital workflows, the field is set to offer even more precise, effective, and patient-centered care. These developments will continue to align with the core principles of minimally invasive dentistry, ensuring that the focus remains on preserving natural tooth structure, reducing patient discomfort, and optimizing clinical outcomes. As these innovations unfold, they will undoubtedly enhance the practice of dentistry and contribute to a more advanced and patient-focused approach to oral health care.

The trajectory of minimally invasive dentistry is increasingly characterized by a focus on enhancing precision, efficiency, and patient-centered care through innovations and emerging technologies. As the field continues to evolve, several critical developments are shaping its future and redefining the boundaries of dental practice.

One area of significant advancement is the integration of artificial intelligence (AI) in diagnostic and treatment planning processes. AI algorithms, powered by machine learning, are becoming proficient at analyzing complex datasets to identify patterns and predict outcomes. In the realm of minimally invasive dentistry, AI applications include advanced imaging analysis, where machine learning models enhance the accuracy of detecting dental caries, fractures, and other conditions. These systems can process vast amounts of data from radiographs and other imaging modalities, providing clinicians with valuable insights and recommendations that facilitate early intervention and more personalized treatment plans.

Additionally, the development of AI-driven treatment planning tools is revolutionizing the way dental procedures are approached. These tools can simulate various treatment scenarios, optimizing plans for the least invasive approaches and predicting potential outcomes based on individual patient data. This integration of AI not only streamlines the planning process but also helps in selecting the most effective minimally invasive techniques tailored to each patient's unique needs.

Advances in biomaterials are also driving innovation in minimally invasive dentistry. Researchers are exploring novel materials that offer improved strength, durability, and biocompatibility. One such advancement is the development of bioactive materials that actively interact with the surrounding tooth structure to promote natural remineralization and enhance the bonding process. These materials are designed to release therapeutic agents that aid in the repair of damaged tissues and support the natural regeneration of tooth structure, further aligning with the principles of minimally invasive care.

Another promising development is the refinement of minimally invasive surgical techniques through the use of advanced lasers and piezoelectric instruments. Laser technology continues to advance, offering new wavelengths and more precise control, which enhances the ability to perform delicate procedures with minimal impact on surrounding tissues. Lasers are increasingly used for soft tissue management, cavity preparation, and even endodontic procedures, providing greater precision and reduced postoperative discomfort.

Piezoelectric instruments, which utilize ultrasonic vibrations to cut bone and soft tissue, are gaining prominence for their ability to perform precise, minimally invasive surgical procedures. These instruments allow for more controlled and atraumatic bone removal, making them particularly valuable in procedures such as implant placement and bone grafting. The use of piezoelectric devices aligns with the goal of minimizing tissue disruption and promoting faster healing.

The integration of digital workflows into dental practices is transforming patient care and clinical efficiency. Digital impressions, CAD/CAM systems, and 3D printing technology are becoming standard in the field, enabling the creation of highly accurate and customized restorations. These technologies facilitate a more efficient and precise approach to restorative procedures, reducing the need for traditional, more invasive methods. For example, digital impressions eliminate the need for conventional molds, enhancing patient comfort and streamlining the process of creating custom crowns, veneers, and other restorations.

Moreover, the application of 3D printing technology is expanding beyond restorations to include the production of surgical guides and orthodontic appliances. These innovations allow for the rapid prototyping of patient-specific devices, enhancing the accuracy and efficiency of both restorative and orthodontic treatments. The ability to quickly produce and adjust these appliances based on digital models contributes to a more personalized and minimally invasive approach to care.

Tele-dentistry is another area poised for growth, driven by advancements in communication technology and remote monitoring tools. Tele-dentistry platforms are evolving to support real-time consultations, remote diagnostics, and patient monitoring. These platforms enable dental professionals to provide care and guidance outside of traditional office visits, offering a convenient option for routine check-ups and follow-up care. As technology advances, tele-dentistry is expected to become increasingly integrated into routine dental practice, providing patients with more accessible and continuous care.

Looking ahead, the future of minimally invasive dentistry will likely be shaped by ongoing research and technological advancements. The continued exploration of regenerative medicine, including stem cell therapy and tissue engineering, holds the potential to revolutionize the treatment of dental conditions by enabling the regeneration of damaged tissues and even whole teeth. Additionally, the development of new materials, enhanced diagnostic tools, and innovative surgical techniques will continue to refine and expand the scope of minimally invasive approaches.

In summary, the future of minimally invasive dentistry is characterized by a convergence of technological advancements and a commitment to patient-centered care. As emerging technologies and innovative materials further enhance the precision, efficiency, and effectiveness of dental treatments, the field will continue to evolve in ways that align with the principles of minimally invasive care. These developments will not only improve patient outcomes but also drive the continued advancement of dental practice, ensuring that minimally invasive dentistry remains at the forefront of modern oral health care.

CHAPTER 29: BUILDING A MINIMALLY INVASIVE DENTAL PRACTICE

Establishing a dental practice centered around minimally invasive techniques requires a thoughtful approach that integrates the latest technologies with a commitment to conservative care. The journey to creating such a practice begins with a thorough understanding of the principles and benefits of minimally invasive dentistry, followed by the careful selection of technologies and the development of workflows that enhance patient outcomes while maximizing practice efficiency.

The foundation of a minimally invasive dental practice is built upon the careful selection of appropriate technologies that align with the principles of conservative care. One of the first steps in this process is to invest in diagnostic tools that provide high-resolution imaging with minimal patient discomfort. Advanced imaging technologies, such as digital radiography and cone-beam computed tomography (CBCT), are essential for accurate diagnosis and treatment planning. Digital radiography offers lower radiation doses compared to traditional film-based methods and provides immediate results that enhance diagnostic capabilities. CBCT, on the other hand, delivers three-dimensional imaging that is invaluable for assessing complex cases and planning procedures with precision.

Another critical component of a minimally invasive practice is the integration of cutting-edge restorative and therapeutic technologies. For instance, the adoption of laser systems can significantly enhance the precision of procedures while minimizing tissue damage and postoperative discomfort. Lasers can be used for a variety of applications, including soft tissue management, cavity preparation, and periodontal treatments. Additionally, the use of CAD/CAM (computer-aided design/computer-aided manufacturing) technology allows for the creation of highly accurate and customized restorations, such as crowns and veneers, which can be fabricated in a single visit, reducing the need for more invasive procedures and multiple appointments.

The design of workflows within a minimally invasive dental practice is another crucial aspect that influences the success of the practice. Workflow optimization involves streamlining processes to enhance efficiency while maintaining a focus on conservative care. This can be achieved by implementing digital systems for patient records, treatment planning, and communication. Electronic health records (EHR) systems facilitate comprehensive and easily accessible patient information, which supports more accurate diagnosis and treatment planning. Furthermore, digital treatment planning tools enable precise simulations of restorative procedures, ensuring that the chosen techniques align with minimally invasive principles.

Patient education and engagement are integral to the success of a minimally invasive practice. Developing effective communication strategies that emphasize the benefits of minimally invasive techniques and the importance of preventive care is essential for fostering a patient-centered approach. This includes educating patients about their treatment options, the rationale behind conservative approaches, and the potential outcomes of different procedures. Providing clear, understandable information helps patients make informed decisions and promotes adherence to recommended preventive measures, which can ultimately reduce the need for more invasive interventions.

Building a team skilled in minimally invasive techniques is essential for the successful implementation of a practice focused on conservative care. This involves not only hiring practitioners with expertise in minimally invasive dentistry but also investing in ongoing training and professional development. Ensuring that all team members are proficient in the latest techniques and technologies supports a cohesive approach to patient care and enhances overall practice performance. Continuing education opportunities, workshops, and professional conferences are valuable resources for keeping the team updated on advancements in minimally invasive dentistry and refining their skills.

Moreover, fostering a collaborative practice environment where team members can share knowledge and best practices is crucial. Regular team meetings and case discussions provide opportunities for practitioners to learn from one another and stay abreast of emerging techniques and technologies. Encouraging an atmosphere of open communication and continuous learning helps maintain high standards of care and supports the successful integration of minimally invasive methods into daily practice.

Patient-centered care extends beyond the treatment room and into the overall practice experience. Creating a welcoming and comfortable environment for patients contributes to a positive experience and reinforces the practice's commitment to minimally invasive principles. This includes implementing practices that reduce patient anxiety, such as offering sedation options for more sensitive procedures and ensuring that the practice environment is calm and reassuring. Additionally, integrating patient feedback mechanisms allows for ongoing improvement and adaptation of services to better meet patient needs and expectations.

In summary, building a minimally invasive dental practice involves a multifaceted approach that includes the careful selection of technologies, the design of efficient workflows, and the development of a skilled and knowledgeable team. By focusing on these key areas, dental practitioners can create a practice that emphasizes conservative care, enhances patient outcomes, and remains at the forefront of modern dental practice. As the field of minimally invasive dentistry continues to evolve, maintaining a commitment to these principles will ensure that the practice remains aligned with the latest advancements and continues to provide exceptional care to patients.

The successful establishment of a minimally invasive dental practice hinges not only on the selection of appropriate technologies and the design of efficient workflows but also on the effective management of patient relationships and the development of a robust operational framework. Building a practice that prioritizes conservative care involves creating a patient experience that aligns with the principles of minimally invasive dentistry while ensuring operational excellence.

The integration of patient-centered care into the operational framework of a minimally invasive dental practice requires a strategic approach to patient management and service delivery. One of the core elements is the development of a comprehensive patient intake and assessment process. This involves gathering detailed patient histories, conducting thorough clinical evaluations, and utilizing advanced diagnostic tools to inform treatment planning. Implementing a patient management system that seamlessly integrates with digital diagnostic tools can streamline these processes, ensuring that patient information is accurately recorded and readily accessible for clinical decision-making.

Incorporating preventive care protocols into the practice is another crucial aspect of aligning with minimally invasive principles. Preventive measures should be embedded into every stage of patient interaction, from initial consultations to routine check-ups. This includes promoting regular dental visits, conducting risk assessments for dental issues, and offering personalized recommendations for home care. Educational materials and interactive tools can be used to engage patients in their oral health, helping them understand the importance of preventive measures and how they contribute to minimizing the need for invasive treatments.

Furthermore, the design of the patient journey within the practice should reflect the principles of minimally invasive care. This involves creating a practice environment that supports a calm and positive patient experience, reducing anxiety and discomfort. The layout of the practice should facilitate easy navigation and accessibility, with clear signage and comfortable waiting areas. The use of patient comfort measures, such as sedation options for anxious patients and the availability of amenities like noise-canceling headphones or relaxing music, can enhance the overall patient experience and contribute to a more positive perception of the practice.

Effective communication is essential in fostering patient trust and ensuring that patients are well-informed about their treatment options. Developing clear and consistent communication strategies, both verbal and written, is key to achieving this goal. This includes providing detailed explanations of treatment procedures, discussing the benefits and limitations of different options, and addressing any concerns or questions that patients may have. Utilizing visual aids, such as digital simulations or educational videos, can further enhance patient understanding and facilitate informed decision-making.

The implementation of feedback mechanisms is another important aspect of building a successful minimally invasive dental practice. Regularly soliciting feedback from patients allows for the continuous evaluation and improvement of practice operations and patient care. This can be achieved through surveys, comment cards, or follow-up communications. Analyzing patient feedback helps identify areas for improvement and provides valuable insights into patient preferences and expectations, enabling the practice to adapt and enhance its services accordingly.

In addition to patient management and care, the operational efficiency of the practice plays a critical role in its overall success. Establishing streamlined administrative processes, including appointment scheduling, billing, and inventory management, can significantly impact the practice's efficiency and profitability. Implementing practice management software that integrates these functions can facilitate seamless operations and reduce administrative burdens. Regular staff training and the development of standardized protocols for common procedures ensure consistency and quality in service delivery.

Financial management is also a crucial component of building a successful minimally invasive practice. Developing a sound financial plan that includes budgeting for technology investments, operational expenses, and staff compensation is essential. Additionally, implementing strategies for revenue generation and cost control can help maintain financial stability and support the long-term growth of the practice. Offering flexible payment options, such as financing plans or payment plans, can also enhance accessibility for patients and increase practice profitability.

Finally, establishing a strong brand identity and marketing strategy is key to attracting and retaining patients. Creating a compelling brand that reflects the values and principles of minimally invasive dentistry can differentiate the practice in a competitive market. This includes developing a professional and engaging online presence, utilizing social media to connect with potential patients, and implementing targeted marketing campaigns that highlight the benefits of minimally invasive techniques. Building a positive reputation through patient testimonials and community involvement further enhances the practice's visibility and appeal.

In summary, building a minimally invasive dental practice requires a multifaceted approach that encompasses patient management, operational efficiency, financial planning, and effective marketing. By focusing on these areas, dental practitioners can create a practice that not only emphasizes conservative care but also delivers a high-quality patient experience and achieves long-term success. The integration of advanced technologies, streamlined workflows, and patient-centered care principles will ensure that the practice remains at the forefront of modern dentistry and continues to meet the evolving needs of patients.

Developing a minimally invasive dental practice also involves a commitment to continuous improvement and adaptation to new advancements. To maintain excellence and relevance in a field that is constantly evolving, dental practitioners must stay abreast of the latest research, technological innovations, and best practices. This commitment requires an ongoing investment in professional development and a culture of learning within the practice.

One essential aspect of fostering a culture of learning is encouraging continuous education for all members of the dental team. This includes not only the dentist but also dental hygienists, dental assistants, and administrative staff. Offering regular training sessions, attending dental conferences, and participating in webinars or online courses ensures that the team is up-to-date with the latest techniques and technologies in minimally invasive dentistry. Professional development should be seen as an integral part of practice growth, as it enhances the team's skills and knowledge, leading to improved patient outcomes and satisfaction.

Integrating new technologies into the practice is another critical factor in maintaining a competitive edge. Emerging technologies such as digital radiography, CAD/CAM systems, and laser dentistry have transformed the landscape of minimally invasive dentistry. These technologies not only improve diagnostic accuracy and treatment precision but also enhance patient comfort and reduce treatment times. Investing in state-of-the-art equipment requires careful consideration of the initial costs, training requirements, and potential return on investment. However, the benefits of incorporating advanced technologies often outweigh the costs by improving practice efficiency and patient care.

In addition to technological advancements, new materials and techniques continually emerge in the field of minimally invasive dentistry. Staying informed about these innovations allows practitioners to offer the most effective and conservative treatments available. For instance, advancements in adhesive technologies and restorative materials can lead to more durable and esthetically pleasing outcomes with less invasive procedures. Implementing these innovations requires evaluating their clinical efficacy, compatibility with existing protocols, and overall impact on patient care.

Building a team that is adept at minimally invasive techniques also involves creating an environment that fosters collaboration and communication. Effective teamwork and open communication among team members are crucial for delivering cohesive and patient-centered care. Regular team meetings, case discussions, and collaborative treatment planning sessions help ensure that all members of the team are aligned with the practice's goals and approach. Encouraging a collaborative culture also facilitates the exchange of knowledge and ideas, which can lead to improved problem-solving and innovation within the practice.

Patient engagement and education remain central to the success of a minimally invasive dental practice. Developing a comprehensive patient education program that explains the benefits of minimally invasive treatments and encourages proactive oral health management can significantly impact patient outcomes. Educational materials, such as brochures, videos, and interactive tools, should be designed to address common patient concerns and misconceptions about minimally invasive dentistry. Personalized education during appointments, where patients can discuss their specific needs and treatment options with their dentist, further reinforces the value of conservative care.

Implementing a robust follow-up system is also essential for ensuring the long-term success of minimally invasive treatments. Regular follow-up appointments allow for the monitoring of treatment outcomes, the management of any issues that arise, and the reinforcement of preventive measures. Developing a system for tracking patient progress and maintaining clear records of treatment plans and outcomes helps identify trends and areas for improvement.

The operational efficiency of a minimally invasive dental practice can be further enhanced by leveraging data and analytics. Utilizing practice management software that offers analytics capabilities can provide valuable insights into practice performance, patient demographics, and treatment outcomes. Analyzing this data helps identify areas where efficiencies can be improved, resources can be better allocated, and patient care can be optimized.

Finally, fostering a positive and supportive work environment contributes to the overall success of the practice. A practice that values and supports its team members is more likely to experience high levels of employee satisfaction and retention. Offering opportunities for career advancement, recognizing and rewarding achievements, and maintaining a healthy work-life balance are all factors that contribute to a positive work environment. When team members are motivated and engaged, they are more likely to provide exceptional care and contribute to the practice's success.

In summary, building a minimally invasive dental practice involves more than just adopting new techniques and technologies. It requires a comprehensive approach that includes investing in continuous education, integrating advanced technologies, fostering a collaborative team environment, engaging patients in their care, and leveraging data for operational improvements. By focusing on these areas, dental practitioners can create a practice that not only excels in delivering minimally invasive care but also achieves long-term success and growth. The commitment to ongoing learning and adaptation ensures that the practice remains at the forefront of modern dentistry and continues to meet the evolving needs of patients.

CHAPTER 30: TRAINING AND PROFESSIONAL DEVELOPMENT IN MINIMALLY INVASIVE DENTISTRY

The evolving landscape of minimally invasive dentistry necessitates a robust framework for training and professional development to ensure that practitioners are adept with the latest techniques and technologies. As the field continues to advance, the importance of continuous education and skill enhancement becomes increasingly evident. This chapter delves into the essential components of training and professional development in minimally invasive dentistry, highlighting the available educational resources, workshops, and advanced training programs designed to keep practitioners current and proficient.

Training in minimally invasive dentistry encompasses a broad spectrum of learning opportunities, from foundational education in dental school to specialized advanced training. Initial exposure to minimally invasive techniques often occurs during dental school, where students are introduced to conservative approaches and the principles of preserving healthy tooth structure. However, the field's rapid development means that the knowledge acquired during formal education requires regular updates and expansions throughout a practitioner's career.

Continuing education plays a pivotal role in maintaining and enhancing professional competence. Various avenues are available for practitioners to access ongoing education, including accredited courses, online webinars, and live workshops. These educational opportunities are designed to address the specific needs of dental professionals by focusing on new techniques, technological advancements, and evidence-based practices in minimally invasive dentistry.

Accredited courses offer structured learning experiences and are often provided by professional dental organizations, universities, and specialized training institutions. These courses typically cover a range of topics, from advanced restorative techniques and laser applications to the latest developments in diagnostic tools. By participating in these courses, practitioners can gain in-depth knowledge and hands-on experience with new methods and technologies, thereby enhancing their ability to implement minimally invasive practices effectively.

Online webinars and virtual learning platforms have become increasingly popular, providing flexibility for practitioners who may not have the time to attend in-person events. These platforms offer a wide array of topics relevant to minimally invasive dentistry and often feature expert speakers who share their insights and experiences. The advantage of online learning lies in its accessibility, allowing practitioners to engage with educational content at their convenience and stay current with the latest developments in the field.

Workshops and hands-on training sessions provide practical,

interactive learning experiences that are crucial for mastering minimally invasive techniques. These workshops are often led by experts in the field and are designed to simulate real-world scenarios, allowing practitioners to practice new skills under the guidance of experienced instructors. The hands-on component of these workshops is particularly valuable, as it enables practitioners to refine their techniques and gain confidence in applying them to patient care.

Advanced training programs are available for those seeking to specialize further or develop expertise in specific areas of minimally invasive dentistry. These programs often involve a more intensive curriculum and may include clinical rotations, research projects, and mentorship opportunities. Advanced training is beneficial for practitioners who wish to incorporate cutting-edge techniques into their practice or take on leadership roles in the field.

Professional development in minimally invasive dentistry also involves staying informed about the latest research and evidence-based practices. Dental journals, research publications, and professional conferences provide valuable resources for practitioners to learn about emerging trends, study results, and new innovations. Engaging with the current literature and participating in research activities help practitioners stay at the forefront of the field and contribute to the ongoing advancement of minimally invasive techniques.

Mentorship and peer collaboration are integral components of professional development. Experienced practitioners can offer guidance and support to less experienced colleagues, sharing their knowledge and insights. Mentorship relationships can provide practical advice, career development support, and a platform for discussing challenging cases and treatment strategies. Peer collaboration through professional networks and dental associations also fosters a community of practice where practitioners can exchange ideas, discuss best practices, and collaborate on research and clinical initiatives.

The commitment to professional development is not only beneficial for individual practitioners but also for the broader dental community. By continuously updating their skills and knowledge, practitioners contribute to the overall advancement of minimally invasive dentistry and help to elevate the standard of care within the field. Furthermore, a well-trained and knowledgeable dental team can improve patient outcomes, enhance patient satisfaction, and drive the successful implementation of minimally invasive techniques in clinical practice.

In summary, training and professional development are crucial for maintaining proficiency and excellence in minimally invasive dentistry. From foundational education to advanced training programs, various resources and opportunities are available to support practitioners in their pursuit of continuous improvement. Engaging in accredited courses, online webinars, workshops, and advanced training, along with staying informed about the latest research and fostering mentorship and peer collaboration, ensures that dental professionals remain at the cutting edge of minimally invasive practices. By prioritizing ongoing education and skill enhancement, practitioners can provide the highest level of care, adapt to new advancements, and contribute to the advancement of minimally invasive dentistry.

The realm of minimally invasive dentistry is dynamic, marked by rapid advancements in techniques, technologies, and materials. Consequently, the need for continuous professional development is paramount for practitioners striving to stay current and provide the highest standard of care. Engaging in ongoing training not only ensures that practitioners are well-versed in the latest methodologies but also fosters a culture of lifelong learning that benefits both patients and the dental community at large.

One critical aspect of professional development is the availability of educational resources tailored to minimally invasive dentistry. These resources include not only textbooks and academic journals but also multimedia materials such as instructional videos and online modules. Textbooks provide foundational knowledge and comprehensive coverage of established techniques, while academic journals offer insights into the latest research findings and evidence-based practices. Multimedia resources, on the other hand, offer visual demonstrations of techniques, which can be particularly beneficial for understanding complex procedures and staying updated on recent innovations.

Workshops are another vital component of professional development. These hands-on sessions allow practitioners to engage directly with new tools and techniques under the guidance of experienced instructors. Workshops often focus on specific areas of minimally invasive dentistry, such as laser application, adhesive dentistry, or digital imaging technologies. The interactive nature of workshops helps practitioners to refine their skills, troubleshoot problems in real-time, and gain practical experience that can be directly applied to their clinical practice. Furthermore, workshops provide an opportunity for networking and collaboration with peers, fostering a sense of community and shared learning among dental professionals.

Advanced training programs represent a more intensive approach to professional development. These programs are designed for practitioners seeking to deepen their expertise or specialize in particular aspects of minimally invasive dentistry. Advanced training often includes a combination of theoretical learning, clinical practice, and research components. For instance, a program might involve coursework on advanced restorative techniques, followed by supervised clinical practice where practitioners apply these techniques in real-world scenarios. Research activities may include evaluating new materials or techniques, contributing to the body of knowledge in the field, and advancing evidence-based practices.

Specialized certifications and fellowships are available for those who wish to demonstrate their expertise and commitment to minimally invasive dentistry. Obtaining certification from reputable organizations can enhance a practitioner's credentials and signal a high level of proficiency to patients and peers alike. Fellowships often involve mentorship, advanced training, and participation in research projects, providing a comprehensive approach to professional development and allowing practitioners to become leaders in the field.

Keeping abreast of technological advancements is another crucial element of professional development. The field of minimally invasive dentistry is characterized by rapid technological progress, including the development of new diagnostic tools, imaging techniques, and treatment materials. Practitioners must stay informed about these advancements to effectively integrate new technologies into their practice. This might involve attending technology-specific seminars, participating in manufacturer-sponsored training sessions, or engaging in online forums and webinars dedicated to technological innovations in dentistry.

Research and evidence-based practice are integral to advancing minimally invasive dentistry. Practitioners should actively engage with the latest research findings, which can provide valuable insights into the efficacy of new techniques and materials. Participation in research activities, whether through clinical trials, observational studies, or collaborative research projects, contributes to the development of best practices and helps to ensure that clinical decisions are grounded in solid evidence. Keeping up with the literature, attending research conferences, and contributing to scholarly publications are essential for practitioners aiming to stay at the forefront of the field.

Mentorship and peer collaboration are also vital components of ongoing professional development. Experienced practitioners can offer guidance and support to less experienced colleagues, sharing their expertise and providing valuable feedback. Mentorship relationships can help newer practitioners navigate complex cases, adopt best practices, and develop their clinical skills. Peer collaboration, through professional associations and networking events, allows practitioners to exchange ideas, discuss challenges, and explore innovative solutions together.

In summary, training and professional development in minimally invasive dentistry are crucial for maintaining clinical excellence and advancing the field. Practitioners must engage in a variety of educational activities, including accessing educational resources, attending workshops, participating in advanced training programs, and staying updated with technological and research advancements. By committing to lifelong learning and professional growth, dental professionals can enhance their skills, provide optimal patient care, and contribute to the continued evolution of minimally invasive dentistry.

The landscape of minimally invasive dentistry is continually evolving, making ongoing training and professional development essential for practitioners who wish to remain at the forefront of their field. As new techniques and technologies emerge, dental professionals must not only become adept at utilizing these innovations but also understand their implications for patient care and practice management.

One significant aspect of continuous professional development is the integration of advanced technological tools into dental practice. For instance, the advent of digital impressions and 3D imaging technologies has revolutionized diagnostic and treatment planning processes. Mastery of these tools requires not just an understanding of their operational aspects but also an appreciation of how they influence treatment outcomes and patient experience. Training programs that focus on the practical application of these technologies help practitioners gain proficiency and confidence, ensuring that they can leverage these tools to enhance the precision and effectiveness of their treatments.

Another crucial component of professional development is the ability to stay informed about the latest research and evidence-based practices. The field of minimally invasive dentistry relies heavily on scientific evidence to guide clinical decisions and validate new approaches. Access to up-to-date research through journals, online databases, and professional conferences is vital for practitioners to make informed decisions and implement best practices. Engaging with the latest studies allows practitioners to understand emerging trends, evaluate new materials and techniques, and apply evidence-based interventions to their practice.

Furthermore, the evolution of minimally invasive techniques often involves the development of new materials and technologies. Staying current with these advancements requires practitioners to engage in specialized training programs and workshops that focus on the latest innovations. For example, the introduction of bioactive materials and advanced adhesive systems necessitates an understanding of their properties, benefits, and limitations. Training sessions that cover these aspects help practitioners incorporate new materials into their practice effectively, optimizing treatment outcomes and patient satisfaction.

Peer collaboration and interdisciplinary learning also play a critical role in professional development. Interactions with colleagues and specialists from related fields can provide valuable insights and broaden a practitioner's perspective on minimally invasive techniques. Collaborative learning environments, such as study groups, online forums, and professional associations, facilitate the exchange of ideas, sharing of experiences, and discussion of complex cases. This collaborative approach not only enhances technical skills but also fosters a deeper understanding of the interdisciplinary aspects of dental care.

Mentorship and coaching are integral to the development of advanced skills and expertise in minimally invasive dentistry. Experienced practitioners who serve as mentors can offer personalized guidance, support, and feedback, helping less experienced colleagues navigate the complexities of advanced techniques and technologies. Mentorship relationships provide an opportunity for skill refinement, problem-solving, and professional growth, contributing to the overall advancement of the field. Additionally, mentoring fosters a culture of knowledge sharing and professional development within the dental community.

The role of professional organizations and certification bodies in supporting continuous development cannot be overlooked. These organizations often provide resources such as accredited continuing education courses, certification programs, and professional guidelines that help practitioners maintain their skills and knowledge. Certification in specific areas of minimally invasive dentistry not only enhances a practitioner's credentials but also demonstrates a commitment to high standards of care and ongoing learning.

Finally, self-directed learning and reflection are essential components of professional growth. Practitioners should regularly assess their skills, review their clinical outcomes, and seek feedback from peers and patients. Reflective practices, such as reviewing case studies, participating in self-assessment exercises, and setting personal learning goals, enable practitioners to identify areas for improvement and develop strategies for enhancing their clinical practice.

In conclusion, training and professional development in minimally invasive dentistry are crucial for maintaining high standards of care and adapting to ongoing advancements in the field. By engaging in a variety of educational activities, staying informed about the latest research and technologies, participating in peer collaboration and mentorship, and pursuing certification and self-directed learning, practitioners can ensure they remain proficient and effective in their practice. This commitment to continuous learning not only benefits individual practitioners but also contributes to the advancement of minimally invasive dentistry as a whole, ultimately leading to improved patient outcomes and enhanced professional satisfaction.

CHAPTER 31: ENHANCING PATIENT EXPERIENCE THROUGH MINIMALLY INVASIVE TECHNIQUES

The patient experience is a critical component of dental care, influencing not only patient satisfaction but also clinical outcomes and practice success. Minimally invasive techniques, with their focus on preserving healthy tissue and reducing the invasiveness of dental procedures, have the potential to significantly enhance patient experience. This chapter explores how these techniques contribute to greater comfort, quicker recovery times, and overall positive experiences for patients, while offering strategies for effectively communicating these benefits.

A fundamental aspect of minimally invasive dentistry is its emphasis on conserving as much healthy tooth structure as possible. Traditional dental procedures often involve significant removal of tooth material, which can lead to discomfort, increased risk of complications, and longer recovery times. In contrast, minimally invasive techniques aim to address dental issues with a conservative approach, resulting in less trauma to the tooth and surrounding tissues. For patients, this translates to reduced pain and discomfort during and after procedures, contributing to a more favorable overall experience.

One of the primary ways minimally invasive techniques enhance patient comfort is through the use of advanced technology. Digital imaging, for example, allows for precise diagnostics with minimal radiation exposure, reducing the need for multiple imaging sessions and associated discomfort. Similarly, air abrasion and laser technology enable more precise removal of decay with less heat and vibration compared to traditional drills, minimizing patient discomfort during the procedure. These technological advancements contribute to a more pleasant experience, as patients experience less noise and pressure, leading to reduced anxiety and stress.

In addition to improved comfort during treatment, minimally invasive techniques often result in quicker recovery times. Traditional dental procedures, particularly those involving extensive drilling and material removal, can leave patients with significant discomfort and a longer healing period. Minimally invasive approaches, however, are designed to be less traumatic, which often leads to faster healing and reduced postoperative pain. This quicker recovery is particularly beneficial for patients with busy schedules or those who are apprehensive about dental procedures, as it allows them to return to their normal activities with minimal disruption.

Effective communication is essential in ensuring that patients understand and appreciate the benefits of minimally invasive techniques. Dental professionals should take the time to explain the nature of the procedures, the reasons for choosing a minimally invasive approach, and the anticipated outcomes. This includes discussing how these techniques can lead to less discomfort, faster recovery, and better long-term results. Providing patients with clear and concise information helps to alleviate their concerns and enhances their confidence in the treatment plan.

Incorporating visual aids can also be beneficial in communicating the advantages of minimally invasive techniques. For example, before-and-after images or diagrams can help patients visualize the benefits of preserving healthy tooth structure and how advanced technologies contribute to a more comfortable experience. Demonstrations of equipment, such as laser devices or air abrasion units, can further reassure patients by showing them how these tools work and how they differ from traditional methods.

Patient education extends beyond the initial consultation and should be an ongoing process. Providing patients with written materials, such as brochures or informational sheets, can reinforce the benefits of minimally invasive techniques and address any questions they may have. Additionally, follow-up appointments offer opportunities to discuss the outcomes of the procedures, address any concerns, and provide additional guidance on post-treatment care. This ongoing support helps to maintain positive patient experiences and build trust between patients and their dental care providers.

It is also important for dental practices to create a welcoming and supportive environment that fosters a positive patient experience. This includes ensuring that the clinical setting is comfortable, maintaining clear and open lines of communication, and offering empathetic and attentive care. Training staff to address patient concerns with sensitivity and professionalism contributes to a supportive atmosphere that enhances the overall experience of care.

Ultimately, the goal of enhancing patient experience through minimally invasive techniques is to improve outcomes and satisfaction while reducing the impact of dental procedures on patients' lives. By focusing on patient comfort, quick recovery, and effective communication, dental professionals can create a more positive and rewarding experience for their patients. The implementation of minimally invasive techniques represents a significant advancement in dental care, and when combined with thoughtful patient engagement, it can lead to a more satisfying and effective practice.

In conclusion, minimally invasive techniques offer significant benefits for enhancing patient experience, including increased comfort, faster recovery, and overall positive outcomes. By adopting these techniques and communicating their advantages effectively, dental professionals can improve patient satisfaction and foster a more positive perception of dental care. This approach not only enhances the quality of care but also contributes to the long-term success and reputation of the dental practice.

Minimally invasive techniques have revolutionized dental practice by prioritizing patient comfort and expediting recovery. These methods inherently reduce the extent of intervention, which has profound implications for the patient experience. Central to this experience is the reduction of discomfort and the acceleration of healing, both of which are vital to patient satisfaction and overall treatment success.

One significant advantage of minimally invasive dentistry is its ability to diminish procedural pain. Traditional dental procedures often involve extensive drilling and tissue removal, which can be accompanied by considerable discomfort. In contrast, minimally invasive approaches utilize advanced technologies such as lasers and air abrasion, which are less invasive and typically result in less pain. Lasers, for instance, can precisely target and remove decay while minimizing damage to surrounding healthy tissue. This targeted approach reduces the need for local anesthesia and the associated discomfort, leading to a more comfortable experience for the patient.

Another benefit of minimally invasive techniques is the potential for reduced anxiety. The prospect of undergoing dental procedures can be daunting for many patients, particularly those who have had negative experiences in the past. Minimally invasive methods often involve less noise and vibration compared to traditional drilling, which can help alleviate some of the anxiety associated with dental visits. The use of quieter, less intimidating tools contributes to a calmer environment, helping to ease patient fears and improve their overall experience.

Recovery times are a critical factor in patient satisfaction. Conventional dental procedures can require extended periods for healing, during which patients may experience pain, swelling, and discomfort. Minimally invasive techniques, by contrast, aim to preserve as much of the healthy tooth structure as possible, resulting in less trauma to the surrounding tissues. This approach not only facilitates quicker healing but also reduces the likelihood of postoperative complications. Patients often find that they can resume their normal activities more quickly, which is a significant advantage in terms of both convenience and comfort.

Effective communication plays a crucial role in enhancing the patient experience with minimally invasive techniques. It is essential for dental professionals to convey the benefits of these approaches clearly and empathetically. During initial consultations, practitioners should take the time to explain how minimally invasive techniques differ from traditional methods and why they are preferable for certain conditions. This includes discussing how these techniques can reduce pain, minimize recovery time, and improve long-term outcomes.

Providing patients with visual aids can further enhance understanding and comfort. For instance, before-and-after images of similar cases or animations demonstrating the procedure can help patients grasp the nature of the intervention and its benefits. Demonstrating the equipment used in minimally invasive procedures can also help demystify the process and alleviate concerns. Seeing the technology in action can reassure patients that their treatment will be less invasive and more comfortable than they might have anticipated.

Patient education should not end with the initial consultation. Continuous engagement throughout the treatment process is essential. Follow-up appointments provide opportunities to address any additional questions or concerns, reinforce the benefits of the chosen techniques, and offer guidance on post-treatment care. Providing educational materials, such as brochures or online resources, can also support patient understanding and contribute to a more positive experience.

Creating a supportive and empathetic practice environment further enhances the patient experience. Staff training should emphasize the importance of addressing patient concerns with sensitivity and professionalism. A friendly and attentive approach helps to build trust and rapport, making patients feel more at ease and valued. Ensuring that the practice is equipped with comfortable facilities and maintaining a clean and welcoming environment also contributes to a positive overall experience.

In addition to enhancing individual patient experiences, integrating minimally invasive techniques into practice can contribute to a broader shift in patient perception of dental care. As patients become more aware of the benefits of these methods, they may be more inclined to seek out dental care proactively rather than postponing it due to fears of discomfort or invasive procedures. This proactive approach can lead to better oral health outcomes and greater overall satisfaction with dental care.

In summary, minimally invasive techniques offer significant advantages in enhancing patient experience by reducing discomfort, minimizing recovery times, and improving overall satisfaction with dental procedures. Through effective communication, patient education, and the creation of a supportive environment, dental professionals can maximize the benefits of these techniques and foster positive patient experiences. By prioritizing patient comfort and employing advanced, less invasive methods, practitioners can significantly improve the quality of care and contribute to a more favorable perception of dental visits.

The success of minimally invasive techniques in enhancing the patient experience extends beyond the immediate procedural advantages to encompass long-term patient management and follow-up care. One crucial aspect is the effective management of patient expectations and experiences post-procedure. Providing clear, detailed instructions on post-treatment care is essential for optimizing recovery and ensuring that patients feel supported throughout the healing process.

Patients often benefit from understanding what to expect after their treatment. This includes guidance on managing any mild discomfort or swelling, recommendations for dietary adjustments, and instructions for oral hygiene maintenance. By offering comprehensive post-treatment care instructions, practitioners can help alleviate any concerns patients may have about their recovery, contributing to a smoother and more comfortable healing experience. Furthermore, addressing potential complications early on can prevent minor issues from escalating, enhancing overall patient satisfaction.

Follow-up care and communication are also integral to maintaining a positive patient experience. Scheduling timely follow-up appointments allows practitioners to monitor healing progress, address any emerging concerns, and reinforce the benefits of the minimally invasive approach. During these visits, practitioners should take the opportunity to discuss the results of the procedure, answer any questions, and provide reassurance. This ongoing engagement demonstrates a commitment to patient care and reinforces the positive impact of the minimally invasive techniques used.

Patient feedback is another valuable tool for enhancing the patient experience. Encouraging patients to share their experiences through surveys or informal conversations can provide insights into areas where the practice excels and identify opportunities for improvement. By actively seeking and addressing patient feedback, practitioners can continuously refine their approaches and ensure that the patient experience remains at the forefront of their practice.

The integration of technology in minimally invasive dentistry also plays a significant role in enhancing patient experience. Advances in digital imaging and diagnostic tools allow for more accurate assessments and treatment planning, reducing the need for invasive procedures. For instance, digital scanners and 3D imaging enable practitioners to create precise models of patients' dental structures, facilitating more accurate and conservative treatments. The ability to visualize and plan treatments with greater precision not only improves outcomes but also enhances patient confidence in the proposed procedures.

Moreover, the use of real-time intraoral cameras during consultations and treatments can further improve patient understanding and comfort. These cameras provide patients with a direct view of their dental conditions and the progress of their treatment. By visually demonstrating the areas of concern and the results of interventions, practitioners can foster greater patient involvement and satisfaction. This transparency helps patients make informed decisions and feel more engaged in their care.

A supportive and empathetic approach by the dental team is also crucial in enhancing the patient experience. Training staff to communicate effectively and empathetically can make a significant difference in how patients perceive their care. Ensuring that all team members, from receptionists to dental hygienists, are attuned to the needs and concerns of patients contributes to a more cohesive and supportive patient experience. Building a practice culture that prioritizes patient-centered care and actively addresses patient concerns can lead to improved patient loyalty and satisfaction.

The broader implications of adopting minimally invasive techniques also reflect positively on the overall patient experience. As practices increasingly embrace these approaches, patients benefit from more personalized and less intrusive care. This shift not only improves individual treatment experiences but also contributes to a more positive perception of dental care as a whole. Patients who experience the benefits of minimally invasive techniques are more likely to advocate for their use and share their positive experiences with others, further enhancing the reputation of the practice.

In conclusion, enhancing the patient experience through minimally invasive techniques involves a multifaceted approach that includes effective communication, comprehensive post-treatment care, ongoing patient engagement, and the integration of advanced technologies. By prioritizing patient comfort and providing supportive, empathetic care, practitioners can significantly improve overall patient satisfaction. The benefits of minimally invasive techniques extend beyond the immediate procedural advantages, contributing to a more positive and rewarding dental care experience that fosters patient trust, engagement, and long-term satisfaction.

CHAPTER 32: ETHICAL CONSIDERATIONS IN MINIMALLY INVASIVE DENTISTRY

In the realm of minimally invasive dentistry, ethical considerations are pivotal in guiding practitioners through the complexities of modern dental care. These considerations encompass a variety of dimensions, including patient consent, the ethical use of advanced technologies, and the balance between innovation and patient welfare.

Patient consent is a fundamental ethical principle in healthcare, and in minimally invasive dentistry, it is crucial for ensuring that patients are well-informed and actively involved in their treatment decisions. The concept of informed consent extends beyond merely obtaining a signature on a consent form; it requires practitioners to engage in meaningful dialogue with patients. This dialogue should encompass a thorough explanation of the proposed treatments, including the benefits, risks, and potential outcomes. Patients must be made aware of the minimally invasive nature of the procedures, how these approaches differ from traditional methods, and the specific advantages they offer.

Effective communication is key to obtaining genuine informed consent. Practitioners should use clear, non-technical language to explain complex procedures and technologies. Visual aids, such as diagrams or digital images, can help patients better understand their condition and the proposed interventions. Additionally, practitioners must address any questions or concerns patients may have, ensuring that they are comfortable with their decisions and fully aware of what to expect. This process not only respects patient autonomy but also fosters a sense of trust and collaboration between the practitioner and patient.

The ethical use of technology in minimally invasive dentistry involves careful consideration of both the benefits and limitations of advanced tools and techniques. While new technologies can enhance diagnostic accuracy and treatment efficacy, they also raise questions about their appropriateness and necessity. Practitioners must assess whether the use of such technologies aligns with the principle of beneficence, which mandates that care should aim to benefit the patient while minimizing harm. This involves evaluating whether the technological advancements genuinely contribute to better patient outcomes or if they might introduce unnecessary risks or complications.

Moreover, the integration of emerging technologies should be approached with caution to avoid potential pitfalls, such as over-reliance on digital tools or the introduction of unnecessary complexity into treatment protocols. Practitioners must remain vigilant about maintaining a balance between technological innovation and patient welfare, ensuring that each technological intervention is used judiciously and with the patient's best interests in mind.

Maintaining high standards of care is another critical ethical consideration in minimally invasive dentistry. As practitioners adopt new techniques and technologies, they must continue to adhere to established standards of care and ensure that their practices align with evidence-based guidelines. This commitment to high standards involves ongoing professional development, rigorous training, and adherence to best practices. Practitioners should continually assess their own proficiency with minimally invasive techniques and seek to enhance their skills through education and practice.

Additionally, ethical practice in minimally invasive dentistry requires transparency and honesty in all interactions with patients. This includes being forthright about the limitations of minimally invasive approaches and acknowledging situations where traditional methods may be more appropriate. Practitioners should avoid any form of misrepresentation or exaggeration of the benefits of minimally invasive techniques, as this can undermine patient trust and lead to ethical breaches.

Balancing innovation with patient welfare is perhaps one of the most challenging ethical dilemmas in minimally invasive dentistry. The drive for innovation must be tempered by a commitment to patient-centered care and the recognition that not all patients will benefit equally from new techniques. Practitioners must carefully consider individual patient needs, preferences, and circumstances when deciding on treatment approaches. This personalized approach ensures that the adoption of new technologies and techniques aligns with each patient's unique situation and promotes optimal outcomes.

The ethical dimension of minimizing harm also plays a significant role in decision-making. Minimally invasive techniques are designed to reduce the impact of dental procedures on patients' well-being, but practitioners must be vigilant about potential risks and complications associated with these approaches. This includes being prepared to manage any adverse effects that may arise and ensuring that patients are informed about potential risks and how they will be addressed.

In summary, ethical considerations in minimally invasive dentistry are multifaceted and integral to delivering high-quality patient care. Practitioners must prioritize informed consent, use technology responsibly, uphold high standards of care, and balance innovation with patient welfare. By adhering to these ethical principles, dental professionals can navigate the complexities of modern dental care while maintaining a commitment to patient-centered practice and ensuring that advancements in minimally invasive techniques enhance, rather than compromise, patient outcomes.

In the context of minimally invasive dentistry, the ethical dimensions extend into several practical and theoretical areas that impact both patient care and professional practice. One of the core ethical challenges is ensuring that technological advancements are employed in ways that genuinely enhance patient outcomes rather than simply showcasing the latest innovations. The ethical use of technology requires that practitioners critically evaluate each technological tool or technique against its ability to deliver real benefits to patients. This scrutiny ensures that the integration of new technologies does not inadvertently compromise patient safety or lead to unnecessary procedures.

An essential aspect of ethical practice involves maintaining a balance between the adoption of new techniques and the preservation of traditional, proven methods. While minimally invasive techniques offer significant advantages, such as reduced recovery times and enhanced patient comfort, they must be used judiciously. Practitioners have a responsibility to discern when these techniques are appropriate and when more traditional approaches might be more effective. This balance is critical to ensuring that patient care remains aligned with the best available evidence and the specific needs of each patient.

Moreover, the ethical principle of non-maleficence, which emphasizes the obligation to "do no harm," plays a significant role in minimally invasive dentistry. This principle requires practitioners to be vigilant about the potential risks associated with new technologies and techniques. Even minimally invasive procedures can carry risks, and it is the responsibility of dental professionals to ensure that these risks are minimized and well-managed. This involves not only careful planning and execution of procedures but also transparent communication with patients about potential risks and uncertainties.

Informed consent is deeply intertwined with the principle of non-maleficence. Practitioners must ensure that patients are not only aware of the benefits of minimally invasive techniques but also fully understand the possible risks and limitations. This comprehensive approach to consent empowers patients to make well-informed decisions about their care. Practitioners should also be prepared to revisit the consent process if there are changes in the treatment plan or if new information emerges about the risks or benefits of the proposed procedures.

Another critical ethical consideration is the need for ongoing professional development and education. As the field of minimally invasive dentistry evolves, practitioners must stay current with the latest advancements and best practices. This commitment to lifelong learning ensures that practitioners can provide the highest standard of care while integrating new techniques and technologies effectively. Continuing education also helps practitioners maintain competency in both traditional and minimally invasive methods, thereby enhancing their ability to offer personalized, evidence-based care.

Ethical practice also involves addressing the broader implications of minimally invasive techniques within the context of public health. While these techniques often improve individual patient outcomes, practitioners must consider their impact on community health and access to care. For instance, the implementation of advanced technologies may be limited by resource availability or disparities in healthcare access. Ensuring equitable access to minimally invasive treatments is an important ethical consideration, as it reflects a commitment to fairness and justice within the healthcare system.

Additionally, the integration of minimally invasive techniques must be aligned with ethical considerations related to cost and resource utilization. While these techniques can offer long-term savings by reducing the need for more invasive procedures, the initial costs of advanced technologies can be substantial. Practitioners must weigh the financial implications of adopting new technologies against their potential benefits to patients. Transparent communication with patients about costs and financial implications is essential to maintaining trust and ensuring that patients can make informed choices about their care.

Ethical considerations also extend to the professional relationships between practitioners and patients. Trust is a fundamental component of the patient-provider relationship, and it is essential that practitioners uphold ethical standards to maintain this trust. This includes being honest about the capabilities and limitations of minimally invasive techniques, avoiding any form of deception or exaggeration about their benefits, and prioritizing the best interests of the patient over personal or financial gain.

In summary, the ethical dimensions of minimally invasive dentistry are multifaceted and integral to delivering high-quality care. Practitioners must navigate the complexities of patient consent, the responsible use of technology, and the balance between innovation and patient welfare. By adhering to ethical principles such as non-maleficence, equity, and transparency, dental professionals can ensure that minimally invasive techniques are used effectively and responsibly, ultimately enhancing patient outcomes and maintaining the integrity of the practice.

Addressing the ethical dimensions of minimally invasive dentistry involves a comprehensive understanding of how to align innovative practices with foundational ethical principles. Central to these considerations is the concept of patient autonomy, which necessitates that patients are given sufficient information to make informed decisions about their care. In minimally invasive dentistry, this means not only explaining the potential benefits and risks associated with new techniques but also contextualizing these in relation to traditional approaches. Providing patients with a balanced view allows them to weigh their options based on a full understanding of their choices, thereby upholding their right to make decisions that best suit their personal needs and values.

Moreover, the ethical use of technology in minimally invasive dentistry extends beyond just the application of new tools and methods. It requires a critical evaluation of the technology's role in improving patient care and its integration into existing treatment protocols. Practitioners must be cautious of adopting technologies that are unproven or not adequately tested. An ethical approach involves rigorous assessment and validation of new tools to ensure that they offer genuine improvements over current practices. This scrutiny helps prevent the misuse of technology driven by marketing hype rather than clinical efficacy, ensuring that patient care remains the primary focus.

Another key ethical issue in minimally invasive dentistry is the potential for over-treatment. The allure of advanced technologies and novel techniques might lead practitioners to recommend treatments that are not necessarily in the best interest of the patient. Over-treatment can occur when new methods are used in situations where traditional, less invasive approaches would suffice. Practitioners must remain vigilant against this tendency and prioritize conservative treatment plans that align with the principles of minimal intervention and patient benefit.

Maintaining high standards of care in the face of rapid technological advancements requires ongoing professional integrity and commitment to evidence-based practice. Practitioners should continuously engage in self-assessment and peer review to ensure their skills and knowledge remain current. This commitment to professional development is essential for maintaining ethical practice in a field that evolves quickly. Continuing education and training not only enhance the practitioner's competence but also contribute to the overall quality of patient care, ensuring that patients benefit from the latest advancements while avoiding potential pitfalls associated with emerging technologies.

Furthermore, ethical considerations in minimally invasive dentistry also encompass the responsible management of patient expectations. Clear and transparent communication about what patients can realistically expect from minimally invasive procedures is crucial. This includes addressing any misconceptions and ensuring that patients understand the limits of what can be achieved with these techniques. Setting realistic expectations helps to foster a trusting relationship between the practitioner and the patient, and it mitigates the risk of dissatisfaction or disillusionment with the outcomes.

In addition to individual patient care, ethical considerations extend to broader practice management and professional conduct. This includes ensuring fair access to minimally invasive treatments and addressing any disparities in care. Practitioners should be mindful of how socioeconomic factors and resource availability can affect patients' access to advanced treatments. Promoting equity in care involves not only offering affordable options but also advocating for policies that support access to quality dental care for all patients, regardless of their financial situation.

The integration of minimally invasive techniques also requires thoughtful consideration of how these practices align with the overall ethical standards of the dental profession. This involves adhering to established guidelines and ethical codes that govern professional behavior. By doing so, practitioners can ensure that their use of minimally invasive techniques is consistent with the values and standards upheld by the broader dental community.

Lastly, ethical considerations must also address the impact of minimally invasive dentistry on the dentist-patient relationship. Building and maintaining trust is essential for effective patient care. Practitioners must engage with patients honestly and empathetically, providing them with the information needed to make informed decisions while respecting their choices. This trust is fundamental to ensuring that patients feel valued and respected throughout their treatment process, which in turn enhances their overall experience and satisfaction with care.

In conclusion, the ethical practice of minimally invasive dentistry requires a careful balance between innovation and patient welfare. By focusing on informed consent, responsible technology use, and maintaining high standards of care, practitioners can navigate the complexities of modern dental practice while upholding the principles of ethical care. This approach ensures that advancements in minimally invasive techniques contribute positively to patient outcomes and the overall integrity of the dental profession.

CHAPTER 33: COLLABORATION AND REFERRALS IN MINIMALLY INVASIVE DENTISTRY

In the realm of minimally invasive dentistry, collaboration and referral networks are vital components that contribute significantly to the holistic management of patient care. As dental practice increasingly adopts techniques that emphasize conservation of natural tooth structure and non-invasive approaches, the need for effective interdisciplinary cooperation becomes ever more apparent. This chapter delves into the intricacies of working with specialists, managing referrals, and ensuring comprehensive care through a network of dental professionals.

The essence of collaboration in minimally invasive dentistry lies in integrating various areas of expertise to deliver patient care that is both comprehensive and finely tuned to individual needs. Minimally invasive techniques often require the involvement of multiple dental specialists, each bringing a unique set of skills to the treatment table. For instance, a patient with complex carious lesions might benefit from the expertise of a restorative dentist skilled in advanced adhesive techniques, while a periodontist's input could be crucial for managing gingival health in conjunction with restorative procedures.

Effective collaboration begins with establishing clear lines of communication among all involved practitioners. This includes not only verbal communication but also the use of shared electronic health records and treatment planning software that enable seamless information exchange. By maintaining comprehensive records and ensuring that all team members have access to the most current patient information, dental professionals can work in concert to develop and implement treatment plans that reflect a unified approach to patient care.

Managing referrals is another critical aspect of effective collaboration. When a general dentist identifies a need for specialized care, the referral process should be executed with precision and clarity. This involves providing specialists with detailed information regarding the patient's history, current condition, and specific treatment goals. A well-structured referral not only streamlines the process but also minimizes the risk of miscommunication or oversight. It is essential for the referring dentist to remain involved throughout the specialist's intervention, ensuring that the patient's care remains cohesive and aligned with the overall treatment objectives.

Incorporating minimally invasive techniques into a collaborative practice requires a nuanced understanding of how these methods intersect with various specialties. For instance, the use of laser technology in carious lesion management may require coordination between restorative dentists and oral surgeons to ensure that the laser treatment integrates smoothly with any necessary surgical interventions. Similarly, the application of minimally invasive orthodontic techniques might necessitate collaboration with periodontists to address potential effects on periodontal health.

Furthermore, fostering a culture of mutual respect and professional development among practitioners can enhance the effectiveness of collaborative efforts. Regular meetings, case discussions, and continuing education opportunities can facilitate knowledge sharing and skill development across the network. This collaborative learning environment helps ensure that all members of the team are up-to-date with the latest advancements in minimally invasive techniques and can apply these innovations to their practice.

The role of patient-centered care in collaboration cannot be overstated. Patients should be kept informed and engaged throughout their treatment journey. Clear communication regarding the roles of different specialists and the rationale behind referrals helps to build trust and alleviate any concerns patients may have about their treatment. Additionally, ensuring that patients understand the benefits of a multidisciplinary approach can enhance their overall experience and satisfaction with their care.

A collaborative approach to minimally invasive dentistry also extends to the management of complex cases that involve multiple treatment modalities. For instance, a patient with extensive dental erosion may require a combination of minimally invasive restorative techniques, dietary counseling, and possibly orthodontic intervention. In such cases, the integration of various specialists' insights ensures that all aspects of the patient's condition are addressed comprehensively and that treatment plans are cohesive and well-coordinated.

Finally, the establishment of referral networks and collaborative relationships should be approached with a long-term perspective. Building trust and effective working relationships with specialists is an ongoing process that requires consistent communication, reliability, and a shared commitment to patient welfare. By cultivating strong professional networks and maintaining open lines of communication, dental practitioners can create an environment where minimally invasive techniques are applied effectively and patient outcomes are optimized.

In conclusion, the integration of collaboration and referral networks within minimally invasive dentistry is essential for delivering comprehensive and effective patient care. Through clear communication, detailed referrals, and a commitment to ongoing professional development, dental practitioners can work together to address complex cases and enhance patient outcomes. By fostering a collaborative practice environment, the field of minimally invasive dentistry can continue to evolve, offering patients the benefits of advanced, coordinated care.

Building upon the foundational principles of collaboration and referral networks in minimally invasive dentistry, it is crucial to delve deeper into the mechanics of effective interdisciplinary cooperation. This involves understanding the roles of various dental specialists, optimizing the referral process, and ensuring that patient care remains cohesive and centered around minimally invasive principles.

Specialists play a pivotal role in the realm of minimally invasive dentistry, each contributing unique skills that enhance overall treatment outcomes. For instance, the role of a periodontist is integral in managing cases where gum health impacts the effectiveness of minimally invasive restorative procedures. Periodontists can provide invaluable insights into the management of periodontal conditions, which, when left untreated, can compromise the success of restorations and other interventions. By collaborating with periodontists, restorative dentists can ensure that their treatments are complemented by appropriate periodontal care, thereby optimizing patient outcomes.

Orthodontists also play a significant role in cases requiring minimally invasive interventions. For patients with malocclusion or other orthodontic issues, orthodontists can offer treatments that align with minimally invasive principles, such as clear aligners or other less invasive orthodontic options. Effective collaboration between orthodontists and general dentists ensures that orthodontic treatments are integrated seamlessly into the patient's overall care plan, minimizing the need for more invasive procedures down the line.

The efficiency of the referral process is crucial in maintaining the integrity of patient care. When referring patients to specialists, it is essential to provide comprehensive and accurate information. This includes detailed documentation of the patient's dental history, the specifics of the condition being addressed, and the proposed treatment plan. Clear and concise referrals facilitate a smooth transition for the patient and ensure that specialists have all necessary information to deliver appropriate care. Moreover, maintaining open lines of communication between referring and receiving practitioners is vital for monitoring patient progress and making necessary adjustments to the treatment plan.

In addition to the practical aspects of referrals, the dynamics of interdisciplinary teamwork must be considered. Establishing effective communication channels and regular updates on patient status can help prevent misunderstandings and ensure that all practitioners are aligned with the treatment goals. This collaborative approach helps to address any issues that may arise promptly, thereby reducing the risk of complications and enhancing the overall efficacy of the treatment plan.

Furthermore, managing patient expectations through effective communication is an essential component of successful interdisciplinary collaboration. Patients must be informed about the roles of various specialists and the reasons for referrals, as well as the benefits of a multidisciplinary approach. Clear communication helps patients understand the rationale behind the treatment plan and fosters a sense of trust and confidence in their care. This is particularly important in minimally invasive dentistry, where patients may be unfamiliar with the benefits and principles of less invasive techniques.

Education and training play a significant role in enhancing collaboration within minimally invasive dentistry. Continuous professional development and education for dental practitioners are essential for staying abreast of the latest advancements and techniques in the field. Workshops, seminars, and advanced training programs offer opportunities for practitioners to learn about new technologies, refine their skills, and engage with specialists in various areas of dentistry. This ongoing education fosters a culture of collaboration and helps practitioners build a network of professionals who are well-versed in minimally invasive practices.

Building and maintaining strong professional relationships with specialists is also a critical aspect of effective collaboration. Trust and mutual respect among practitioners contribute to a positive working environment and facilitate more effective teamwork. Regular case discussions, joint treatment planning sessions, and collaborative decision-making can strengthen these relationships and improve the quality of patient care.

In summary, the successful integration of collaboration and referral networks in minimally invasive dentistry hinges on several key factors: clear communication, comprehensive referrals, effective teamwork, and ongoing professional development. By understanding the roles of various specialists, optimizing the referral process, and fostering strong professional relationships, dental practitioners can enhance patient care and achieve better outcomes through a collaborative approach. This holistic method ensures that minimally invasive techniques are applied effectively and that patients receive the comprehensive, patient-centered care that is at the heart of modern dental practice.

To ensure that collaboration and referrals within minimally invasive dentistry are both effective and beneficial, it is essential to examine the strategic integration of different dental specialties and their impact on patient care. Emphasizing the coordination between various dental professionals, including general dentists, specialists, and allied health providers, can significantly enhance the outcomes of minimally invasive procedures and improve the overall patient experience.

Effective management of referrals begins with the establishment of clear protocols and systems within the practice. A structured referral process not only streamlines patient transitions between practitioners but also ensures that each specialist is equipped with the necessary information to provide optimal care. This involves creating a standardized referral template that captures all relevant clinical details, including diagnostic findings, treatment history, and specific concerns or goals. Such templates facilitate a comprehensive understanding of the patient's condition and enable specialists to tailor their interventions more precisely to the patient's needs.

Moreover, integrating electronic health records (EHR) systems can greatly enhance the efficiency and accuracy of the referral process. EHRs enable seamless sharing of patient information among different practitioners, ensuring that all involved parties have access to up-to-date and accurate data. This integration supports real-time updates and facilitates coordinated care, reducing the risk of redundant tests or conflicting treatment plans. Additionally, EHRs can track referral outcomes and follow-up appointments, providing valuable insights into the effectiveness of the referral process and identifying areas for improvement.

Building strong relationships with specialists and other dental professionals is critical for fostering a collaborative environment. This relationship is often nurtured through regular communication and joint case discussions. Regular meetings or consultations where practitioners review complex cases, share insights, and discuss treatment strategies can lead to more cohesive care planning. These interactions not only enhance mutual understanding but also build trust among practitioners, which is essential for effective collaboration.

Patient-centered communication is a cornerstone of successful collaboration in minimally invasive dentistry. Ensuring that patients are well-informed about the reasons for referrals and the roles of different specialists helps in setting realistic expectations and fostering trust in the multidisciplinary approach. Clear, empathetic communication about the benefits of collaborative care, such as how each specialist contributes to achieving the best outcomes, can alleviate patient concerns and promote adherence to treatment plans.

The role of patient education cannot be overstated. Educating patients about minimally invasive techniques and their benefits, such as reduced discomfort and faster recovery times, can lead to more informed and engaged patients. This education should extend to explaining the collaborative nature of their care, highlighting how each specialist's expertise contributes to their overall treatment. Providing educational materials, such as brochures or digital resources, and engaging in open discussions during consultations can enhance patient understanding and satisfaction.

Continuing professional development for dental practitioners is another essential component of effective collaboration. Staying current with the latest advancements in minimally invasive techniques and technologies through ongoing education helps practitioners integrate new methods and technologies into their practice. Workshops, seminars, and advanced training programs offer opportunities for learning about emerging trends and best practices, which can be shared with colleagues to foster a culture of continuous improvement and innovation.

Creating a culture of collaboration within a dental practice involves more than just procedural changes; it requires a shift in mindset towards a team-oriented approach. Encouraging a collaborative culture begins with leadership setting the tone for teamwork and mutual respect. Practices that prioritize open communication, shared goals, and collective problem-solving are more likely to see the benefits of effective collaboration and improved patient outcomes.

In addition to fostering internal collaboration, engaging in professional networks and associations can provide valuable opportunities for expanding referral networks and staying informed about best practices in minimally invasive dentistry. Participation in professional organizations and attending industry conferences can facilitate connections with other practitioners and specialists, offering a platform for exchanging knowledge and experiences.

In conclusion, enhancing collaboration and referral networks in minimally invasive dentistry requires a multifaceted approach that includes efficient referral management, strong professional relationships, effective patient communication, and ongoing professional development. By implementing structured referral processes, leveraging technology, and fostering a collaborative culture, dental practitioners can ensure comprehensive and cohesive patient care. This integrative approach not only improves the efficacy of minimally invasive techniques but also enhances the overall patient experience, aligning with the principles of modern, patient-centered dental practice.

CHAPTER 34: MANAGING PATIENT EXPECTATIONS IN MINIMALLY INVASIVE TREATMENTS

In minimally invasive dentistry, managing patient expectations is pivotal to achieving both successful outcomes and high levels of patient satisfaction. The nature of minimally invasive treatments often leads to misconceptions about their limitations and potential results. As such, addressing these challenges effectively requires a nuanced approach to communication, goal-setting, and patient education.

Setting realistic treatment goals is foundational in aligning patient expectations with clinical realities. Minimally invasive techniques, while offering significant benefits such as reduced discomfort and faster recovery times, may not always meet every patient's ideal outcomes. It is essential to establish clear, achievable goals from the outset. This process begins with an in-depth assessment of the patient's condition, followed by a discussion of what minimally invasive approaches can realistically accomplish. By defining the scope and limitations of the proposed treatments, practitioners can help patients form a more accurate understanding of what to expect.

Effective communication is a crucial component in managing expectations. During consultations, it is important to use clear and straightforward language, avoiding overly technical jargon that may confuse or mislead patients. Visual aids, such as diagrams or digital simulations, can be invaluable in illustrating the expected outcomes of different treatment options. For instance, before-and-after images or models demonstrating the potential results of a procedure can help patients visualize the benefits and limitations of minimally invasive techniques.

Additionally, addressing patient concerns and questions openly and empathetically can prevent misunderstandings and build trust. Patients who feel heard and understood are more likely to be receptive to realistic discussions about their treatment options. Providing thorough explanations about the nature of the procedure, the expected recovery process, and potential risks ensures that patients have a well-rounded view of their treatment plan.

One of the significant challenges in managing expectations is dealing with situations where patient expectations may not align with clinical realities. This misalignment can arise from a variety of sources, including previous experiences with dental care, misinformation from non-professional sources, or personal ideals about the outcomes of treatment. In such cases, it is crucial to address discrepancies in a manner that is both respectful and informative.

When confronting unrealistic expectations, practitioners should first acknowledge the patient's concerns and validate their feelings. This approach helps maintain a positive rapport and sets the stage for a constructive conversation about the limitations of the treatment. Next, it is important to provide a clear, evidence-based explanation of why certain expectations may not be feasible. This could involve discussing the technical limitations of the procedure, the variability of individual responses to treatment, or the inherent nature of dental conditions that may affect outcomes.

It is also beneficial to offer alternative solutions or compromises when possible. If a patient's expectations exceed what minimally invasive techniques can achieve, suggesting additional or adjunctive treatments that align more closely with their goals can help bridge the gap between expectation and reality. For example, if a patient seeks more dramatic aesthetic improvements than minimally invasive techniques can provide, discussing complementary cosmetic procedures or follow-up treatments might be appropriate.

Setting the stage for ongoing communication is another vital aspect of managing expectations. Encouraging patients to ask questions throughout the treatment process and providing regular updates can help maintain alignment between expectations and actual outcomes. Post-treatment follow-ups should include discussions about the results, any observed variations from expected outcomes, and additional steps if necessary. These follow-ups not only reassure patients but also provide an opportunity to address any emerging concerns or misconceptions.

In summary, managing patient expectations in minimally invasive dentistry involves a comprehensive approach to communication, goal-setting, and patient education. By setting realistic treatment goals, utilizing clear and effective communication strategies, and addressing discrepancies with empathy and evidence-based explanations, practitioners can enhance patient satisfaction and treatment success. This proactive management of expectations ensures that patients are well-informed and prepared for their dental care journey, ultimately contributing to a more positive overall experience in minimally invasive treatments.

Managing patient expectations in minimally invasive treatments also involves addressing psychological and emotional aspects that can influence how patients perceive and react to their care. Psychological readiness and emotional responses can significantly impact a patient's satisfaction and perceived success of a treatment. Therefore, understanding and navigating these factors are crucial components of expectation management.

Patients often come into minimally invasive treatments with varying degrees of anxiety, hope, or skepticism. This emotional state can shape their expectations and reactions to the outcomes. Practitioners need to be sensitive to these emotions and address them thoughtfully. For instance, anxiety about the procedure can lead to heightened concerns about potential outcomes. In such cases, providing reassurance through detailed explanations and demonstrating empathy can help alleviate fears and set a more realistic outlook. Employing calming techniques and discussing what patients can expect before, during, and after the procedure can also play a role in managing anxiety and setting appropriate expectations.

On the other hand, patients who have high hopes for dramatic changes may struggle to accept the more modest improvements that minimally invasive techniques typically offer. In these cases, setting realistic expectations becomes not only a matter of clinical accuracy but also one of managing patient hopes and aspirations. Clear, open conversations about what the techniques can achieve, coupled with a focus on the positive aspects of these methods—such as reduced invasiveness and quicker recovery times—can help balance expectations. It is also beneficial to emphasize the incremental nature of many minimally invasive treatments, which often involve a series of steps or follow-up procedures to achieve the desired result. This perspective helps patients understand that significant improvements may be gradual and requires patience.

Furthermore, integrating patient feedback into the treatment process can be an effective strategy for managing expectations. Regularly soliciting feedback from patients allows practitioners to gauge how well the treatment aligns with their expectations and address any concerns that may arise. This ongoing dialogue helps ensure that any discrepancies between expected and actual outcomes are identified and addressed promptly. It also provides an opportunity for practitioners to adjust treatment plans or expectations as needed, based on real-time feedback.

Another key aspect of managing patient expectations involves educating patients about the role of their own behaviors and compliance in achieving optimal outcomes. Patients should be informed about how factors such as oral hygiene, lifestyle choices, and adherence to post-treatment care instructions can influence the success of minimally invasive treatments. By highlighting the importance of these factors, practitioners can encourage patients to actively participate in their own care and manage their expectations more effectively. Educating patients about their role in the treatment process empowers them to take ownership of their oral health, which can contribute to better outcomes and greater satisfaction.

Effective management of patient expectations also requires addressing potential disappointments or complications in a constructive manner. If a patient's treatment does not yield the expected results, it is essential to approach the situation with transparency and a problem-solving mindset. Discussing the reasons for any deviations from expected outcomes, exploring possible solutions or adjustments, and providing ongoing support can help maintain patient trust and satisfaction. Offering additional treatments or modifications to the original plan can also demonstrate a commitment to achieving the best possible outcome for the patient.

In conclusion, managing patient expectations in minimally invasive dentistry is a multifaceted challenge that involves more than just setting realistic goals and communicating effectively. It encompasses understanding and addressing the psychological and emotional aspects of patient care, integrating feedback into the treatment process, educating patients about their role in achieving outcomes, and handling potential disappointments with transparency and support. By adopting a comprehensive approach to expectation management, practitioners can enhance patient satisfaction, foster positive treatment experiences, and ultimately contribute to the success of minimally invasive dental procedures.

To effectively manage patient expectations in minimally invasive treatments, it is crucial for dental practitioners to implement strategies that not only address the clinical aspects of treatment but also engage patients in an ongoing dialogue about their care. This engagement involves fostering an environment where patients feel heard, respected, and involved in their treatment journey.

A fundamental aspect of this engagement is ensuring that patients have a clear understanding of their treatment options and the expected outcomes associated with each. This can be achieved through comprehensive and transparent discussions during initial consultations. Practitioners should present information in a manner that is both accessible and detailed, avoiding overly technical jargon that might confuse or overwhelm patients. Using visual aids, such as diagrams or models, can also help clarify complex concepts and provide a tangible representation of what the patient might expect.

Moreover, it is important to emphasize that minimally invasive procedures, while designed to be less disruptive and more conservative, do not guarantee instantaneous or dramatic results. By setting realistic expectations from the outset, practitioners can help patients understand that the benefits of such techniques often accrue over time and may require multiple visits or follow-up care. This incremental approach should be communicated clearly, with an emphasis on the overall value and long-term benefits of preserving as much of the natural tooth structure as possible.

In addition to discussing treatment options, practitioners should also address potential risks and limitations of minimally invasive techniques. This involves being honest about what the procedures can and cannot achieve, and preparing patients for possible variations in outcomes. Clear communication about the risks of treatment failure or complications, even if they are rare, ensures that patients are fully informed and can make decisions with a realistic understanding of their potential impact.

Another critical element in managing patient expectations is establishing a strong follow-up care system. Post-treatment care is essential for monitoring progress and addressing any concerns that may arise. Regular follow-up appointments provide opportunities to assess the effectiveness of the treatment, make necessary adjustments, and reinforce the patient's role in maintaining their oral health. During these visits, practitioners should continue to provide feedback, discuss any changes in the patient's condition, and adjust expectations as needed based on their response to the treatment.

Handling situations where patient expectations do not align with clinical realities requires a delicate balance of empathy and professionalism. When discrepancies between expected and actual outcomes occur, it is essential to approach the situation with a solution-oriented mindset. Practitioners should engage in open and honest conversations with patients about the factors that may have contributed to the outcome, and discuss possible next steps or alternative treatments. This approach not only helps address any dissatisfaction but also reinforces the practitioner's commitment to the patient's well-being and satisfaction.

It is also beneficial to involve patients in the decision-making process by actively seeking their input and preferences. This collaborative approach helps align the treatment plan with the patient's personal goals and expectations, and fosters a sense of ownership and engagement in their care. By addressing patient concerns and preferences, practitioners can create a more personalized treatment experience that enhances satisfaction and supports better outcomes.

Additionally, practitioners should be proactive in managing expectations by providing educational resources and support materials that patients can refer to outside of appointments. This can include written instructions, online resources, or referrals to support groups. Providing patients with access to these resources helps reinforce the information discussed during consultations and supports their understanding of the treatment process and expected outcomes.

In summary, managing patient expectations in minimally invasive dentistry involves a comprehensive approach that integrates clear communication, realistic goal setting, and ongoing support. By educating patients about their treatment options, addressing potential risks and limitations, and involving them in their care decisions, practitioners can effectively align expectations with clinical realities. Regular follow-up care and a proactive approach to handling discrepancies further contribute to a positive patient experience and foster trust and satisfaction in the treatment process. This holistic approach not only enhances patient outcomes but also strengthens the practitioner-patient relationship, leading to more successful and fulfilling dental care experiences.

CHAPTER 35: THE IMPACT OF MINIMALLY INVASIVE DENTISTRY ON ORAL HEALTH OUTCOMES

The evolution of minimally invasive dentistry represents a significant paradigm shift in the approach to oral health care. This shift emphasizes preserving tooth structure, preventing disease progression, and improving overall patient outcomes. Understanding the impact of these techniques on oral health requires a comprehensive examination of their benefits, implications for disease prevention, and enhancement of patient satisfaction.

Minimally invasive dentistry is rooted in the principle of conserving as much natural tooth structure as possible while effectively addressing dental issues. This approach contrasts with traditional methods that often involve more extensive removal of healthy tooth material. By prioritizing preservation, minimally invasive techniques not only maintain the integrity of the tooth but also contribute to more favorable long-term oral health outcomes. The fundamental benefit of this approach is its ability to reduce the need for more invasive procedures, which can lead to increased tooth sensitivity, structural compromise, and a greater likelihood of subsequent dental issues.

One of the primary benefits of minimally invasive techniques is their role in early disease detection and intervention. Techniques such as digital imaging and laser diagnostics enable practitioners to identify dental issues at their nascent stages, often before they manifest as significant clinical problems. Early detection facilitates prompt treatment, which can effectively halt the progression of conditions such as carious lesions or periodontal disease. By addressing these issues before they escalate, minimally invasive dentistry helps to preserve tooth structure and prevent more extensive damage that might necessitate complex restorative procedures.

Additionally, minimally invasive techniques contribute to improved preventive care, a cornerstone of modern dental practice. For example, the use of fluoride varnishes, sealants, and remineralization therapies are integral to a preventive strategy that minimizes the risk of caries development and progression. These approaches work by enhancing the natural defense mechanisms of the teeth and inhibiting the growth of harmful bacteria. The application of these preventive measures is less invasive and often more comfortable for patients compared to traditional restorative treatments, thereby encouraging greater patient compliance and better long-term outcomes.

The emphasis on conservative treatment not only benefits individual patients but also contributes to broader public health outcomes. By reducing the incidence of severe dental issues, minimally invasive practices help alleviate the overall burden on dental care systems. This approach can lead to a decrease in the need for complex, costly procedures and reduce the frequency of dental visits required for managing advanced conditions. Consequently, the resources saved can be redirected towards preventive initiatives and education, further enhancing community oral health.

In terms of patient satisfaction, minimally invasive techniques have demonstrated a positive impact. Patients often experience less discomfort and shorter recovery times with these approaches compared to traditional methods. The reduced invasiveness translates to fewer complications and a more pleasant treatment experience, which can significantly influence a patient's perception of their care. Moreover, the conservation of natural tooth structure tends to result in more aesthetically pleasing outcomes, which is an important consideration for many patients seeking dental treatment. By aligning treatment outcomes with patient expectations and preferences, minimally invasive techniques enhance overall satisfaction and foster a positive relationship between patients and their dental providers.

The long-term benefits of minimally invasive dentistry are also evident in the reduced likelihood of future dental problems. By preserving natural tooth structure and addressing issues at their inception, these techniques help to maintain the structural integrity of the teeth. This preservation reduces the need for subsequent interventions and extends the longevity of the natural dentition. Furthermore, the focus on prevention and early intervention helps to mitigate the risk of developing secondary complications, such as root canal infections or tooth fractures, which can occur as a result of extensive restorative work.

Overall, the impact of minimally invasive dentistry on oral health outcomes is profound and multifaceted. By emphasizing tooth preservation, early detection, and preventive care, these techniques contribute to improved long-term dental health and patient satisfaction. The benefits extend beyond individual patients to the broader community, reflecting a shift towards a more sustainable and patient-centered approach to dental care. As the field continues to evolve, ongoing research and advancements will further enhance the effectiveness and accessibility of minimally invasive techniques, solidifying their role in optimizing oral health outcomes and advancing the practice of dentistry.

The application of minimally invasive dentistry (MID) has led to significant advancements in how oral health is managed and maintained. Its impact is evident in various aspects of dental care, particularly in the realms of disease prevention, long-term health outcomes, and patient satisfaction. By focusing on less intrusive methods, MID has reshaped conventional dental practices, aligning them more closely with contemporary needs for both effectiveness and patient comfort.

One of the central tenets of minimally invasive dentistry is its focus on disease prevention rather than treatment of advanced conditions. This proactive approach significantly alters the trajectory of dental health. Techniques such as early caries detection using advanced imaging technologies and diagnostic tools allow practitioners to address potential problems before they develop into more severe issues. The early intervention afforded by these technologies enables the application of preventive measures that can halt or reverse the progression of dental caries and other oral health conditions. For example, the use of resin infiltration can be employed to address incipient carious lesions, effectively arresting their development and thereby avoiding more extensive restorative procedures in the future. This shift towards preventive care aligns with broader public health goals of reducing disease incidence and improving overall health outcomes.

The emphasis on less invasive procedures also contributes to improved long-term oral health. By preserving more of the natural tooth structure and minimizing the removal of healthy tissue, MID techniques enhance the durability and longevity of dental restorations. For instance, in restorative dentistry, conservative approaches such as partial crowns or onlays can often be used instead of full crowns, which traditionally required more extensive tooth preparation. This conservation of natural tooth structure not only maintains the strength and functionality of the tooth but also reduces the likelihood of future complications, such as secondary caries or tooth fractures. Consequently, patients experience fewer instances of restorative failure and enjoy greater overall oral health stability.

Another critical advantage of minimally invasive techniques is their positive effect on patient comfort and recovery. Traditional dental procedures, often involving extensive drilling or surgical interventions, can be associated with significant discomfort and prolonged recovery periods. In contrast, minimally invasive procedures typically involve less trauma to the oral tissues, resulting in reduced postoperative pain, shorter recovery times, and a lower risk of complications. For example, the use of laser technology in soft tissue management can significantly decrease bleeding and discomfort compared to conventional surgical methods. This improved comfort enhances the overall patient experience and can lead to higher levels of patient satisfaction.

Patient satisfaction is a crucial component of the success of any dental practice. Minimally invasive techniques, by virtue of their reduced invasiveness and enhanced comfort, often lead to more positive patient experiences. When patients are less anxious about their procedures and experience fewer adverse effects, their overall perception of care improves. Additionally, the aesthetic outcomes of minimally invasive treatments, such as tooth-colored fillings or veneers, can be more satisfactory to patients compared to traditional metal restorations. This alignment with patient expectations not only improves satisfaction but also fosters trust and loyalty to the dental practice.

Minimally invasive dentistry also influences patient compliance with recommended oral health practices. When patients experience less discomfort and see positive results from conservative treatments, they are more likely to adhere to preventive care recommendations and follow-up visits. This enhanced compliance can further contribute to better long-term oral health outcomes, as patients are more engaged in maintaining their oral hygiene and attending regular check-ups.

Furthermore, the broader implications of minimally invasive techniques extend to healthcare systems as well. By reducing the need for more extensive procedures and associated complications, MID can lower the overall cost of dental care. Fewer complex interventions and reduced incidence of dental emergencies result in cost savings for both patients and healthcare providers. These savings can be redirected towards further preventive measures and educational initiatives, amplifying the positive impact on public oral health.

In summary, the influence of minimally invasive dentistry on oral health outcomes is profound and multifaceted. Its emphasis on prevention, preservation, and patient comfort addresses many of the limitations associated with traditional dental practices. By improving early detection, reducing the need for extensive interventions, enhancing patient satisfaction, and contributing to cost savings, minimally invasive techniques represent a significant advancement in the field of dentistry. As research continues to evolve and new technologies emerge, the potential for even greater improvements in oral health outcomes will likely expand, solidifying the role of minimally invasive dentistry as a cornerstone of modern dental care.

The impact of minimally invasive dentistry (MID) on oral health outcomes extends beyond immediate clinical benefits, influencing long-term patient well-being and the broader scope of dental practice. The paradigm shift towards minimally invasive techniques reflects a deeper understanding of dental health dynamics and patient-centered care, underscoring its significant contributions to improving overall health outcomes.

A critical aspect of minimally invasive dentistry is its role in altering the traditional approach to dental treatment and prevention. By emphasizing early detection and intervention, MID techniques allow for more precise and targeted treatment plans. This shift from reactive to proactive care helps mitigate the risk of disease progression and reduces the need for more invasive procedures. For instance, the use of advanced diagnostic tools such as digital radiography and transillumination enables clinicians to detect carious lesions at a much earlier stage than conventional methods. These technologies allow for interventions that are less disruptive to the tooth structure, preserving more of the natural dentition and thus contributing to better long-term oral health.

Moreover, the focus on conservative treatment approaches in MID aligns with the principle of minimally disruptive care. Techniques such as air abrasion and laser dentistry, which minimize the removal of healthy tooth structure, demonstrate a commitment to preserving the integrity of the natural tooth. This preservation not only enhances the longevity of dental restorations but also reduces the likelihood of future complications. For example, when less tooth structure is removed, the remaining tooth is better able to withstand stress and potential future issues, leading to fewer instances of restorative failures or the need for additional interventions.

The emphasis on patient comfort and reduced recovery times associated with minimally invasive techniques further supports improved oral health outcomes. Traditional dental procedures often involve significant postoperative discomfort and longer recovery periods, which can discourage patients from seeking necessary care. In contrast, minimally invasive techniques typically result in less trauma to oral tissues, translating to reduced pain and faster healing. This enhanced comfort encourages patients to adhere to their treatment plans and follow-up appointments, fostering better overall oral health management.

In addition to individual benefits, minimally invasive dentistry also contributes to public health on a larger scale. Preventive measures such as fluoride treatments and sealants, which are integral to MID, play a crucial role in reducing the incidence of dental caries and other oral diseases. By focusing on prevention and early intervention, these techniques help alleviate the burden of dental diseases on healthcare systems and contribute to improved population health outcomes. Furthermore, the cost-effectiveness of minimally invasive techniques, due to their potential to reduce the need for extensive and costly treatments, represents a significant advantage. The economic benefits are not only evident in reduced patient expenses but also in the more efficient allocation of healthcare resources.

The integration of minimally invasive dentistry into routine practice also reflects a broader trend towards holistic and patient-centered care. By prioritizing techniques that are less invasive and more aligned with patient comfort, dental practitioners are able to offer care that is both effective and empathetic. This alignment with patient values and preferences enhances the overall patient experience, leading to greater satisfaction and improved adherence to preventive and therapeutic recommendations.

As minimally invasive techniques continue to evolve, their impact on oral health outcomes is likely to grow. Innovations in technology, materials, and methodologies will further enhance the precision and effectiveness of MID approaches.

For example, advancements in biomaterials and regenerative techniques hold promise for even more effective preservation of natural tooth structure and improved outcomes for patients. Additionally, ongoing research into the long-term effects of minimally invasive treatments will provide valuable insights into their efficacy and further validate their benefits.

In summary, the impact of minimally invasive dentistry on oral health outcomes is profound and multifaceted. By shifting the focus from invasive procedures to preventive and conservative techniques, MID enhances the quality and longevity of dental care. The benefits of improved disease prevention, better preservation of natural tooth structure, reduced patient discomfort, and greater public health impact underscore the significant contributions of MID to overall dental health. As the field continues to advance, the ongoing refinement of minimally invasive techniques will likely yield even greater improvements in patient outcomes, solidifying the role of MID as a cornerstone of modern dental practice.

CHAPTER 36: MINIMALLY INVASIVE TECHNIQUES IN GERIATRIC DENTISTRY

In the realm of geriatric dentistry, minimally invasive techniques have emerged as pivotal in addressing the unique and often complex dental needs of older adults. As the population ages, the prevalence of dental issues among geriatric patients has increased, necessitating a shift towards methods that prioritize preservation of natural tooth structure and enhance patient comfort. This chapter delves into how minimally invasive approaches are applied in geriatric dentistry, examining their role in managing age-related dental conditions and improving the overall effectiveness of dental care for the elderly.

The aging process brings about a range of changes in oral health that require specialized attention. One of the most prevalent issues is the increased susceptibility to caries and root decay, largely due to a combination of factors such as reduced saliva production, changes in dietary habits, and diminished oral hygiene practices. Moreover, the natural wear and tear of teeth, along with the presence of restorative materials that may degrade over time, can further complicate dental health in older adults. Minimally invasive techniques offer significant advantages in managing these conditions by emphasizing early detection, conservative treatment, and maintenance of oral health.

Early detection of dental issues is crucial for effective management, especially in geriatric patients who may present with subtle or atypical symptoms. Advanced diagnostic tools such as digital radiography and intraoral cameras are instrumental in identifying early signs of carious lesions, cracks, and other dental problems before they escalate. For instance, digital radiography provides high-resolution images with reduced radiation exposure, enabling clinicians to detect carious lesions at their incipient stages. This early intervention aligns with the minimally invasive philosophy by allowing for less aggressive treatments that conserve more of the natural tooth structure.

Another significant consideration in geriatric dentistry is the management of root caries. Root caries are increasingly common among older adults due to gum recession and exposure of the tooth roots. Minimally invasive treatments such as fluoride varnishes and sealants play a crucial role in preventing and managing root caries by enhancing the remineralization process and protecting the exposed areas. Fluoride treatments, for example, are effective in reducing the progression of carious lesions and strengthening the remaining tooth structure. Similarly, sealants can be applied to vulnerable areas to provide a protective barrier against plaque accumulation and bacterial invasion.

Geriatric patients often face challenges related to restorative treatments, including issues with existing restorations and the need for new ones. Traditional restorative techniques may not always be suitable due to factors such as diminished tooth structure, changes in oral environment, and increased risk of complications. Minimally invasive restorative options, such as adhesive dentistry and minimally invasive crowns, provide effective alternatives by focusing on preserving as much natural tooth structure as possible. Adhesive techniques, which use bonding agents to securely attach restorative materials to the tooth, can be particularly beneficial in geriatric patients as they offer a conservative approach that minimizes the need for extensive tooth preparation.

The management of periodontal health is another critical aspect of geriatric dental care. Periodontal disease is prevalent among older adults and can significantly impact oral health if left untreated. Minimally invasive periodontal therapies, such as scaling and root planing combined with adjunctive antimicrobial treatments, help manage periodontal disease while minimizing patient discomfort and promoting faster recovery. The use of ultrasonic scalers and laser therapy has revolutionized periodontal treatment by providing more precise and less invasive options for cleaning and decontaminating periodontal pockets.

Comfort and patient-centered care are fundamental considerations in treating older adults, who may be more sensitive to pain and less tolerant of traditional dental procedures. Minimally invasive techniques, which prioritize gentle handling and reduced intervention, align well with the needs of geriatric patients. For example, the use of laser technology in procedures such as soft tissue management and carious tissue removal reduces the need for drills and minimizes postoperative discomfort. Additionally, sedation options and pain management strategies tailored to the needs of older patients enhance the overall experience and ensure that treatments are both effective and well-tolerated.

Incorporating minimally invasive techniques into geriatric dentistry also requires a comprehensive approach that addresses the broader aspects of patient care. This includes coordinating with other healthcare providers to manage systemic conditions that may impact oral health, such as diabetes and cardiovascular disease. By integrating minimally invasive methods with a holistic approach to patient care, dental professionals can provide more effective and compassionate treatment tailored to the specific needs of older adults.

In summary, the application of minimally invasive techniques in geriatric dentistry represents a significant advancement in the field, offering numerous benefits for managing age-related dental issues. By emphasizing early detection, conservative treatment, and patient comfort, these approaches contribute to improved oral health outcomes and enhance the quality of care for older adults. As the population continues to age, the ongoing development and integration of minimally invasive techniques will play a crucial role in addressing the evolving challenges of geriatric dentistry and ensuring that older patients receive the highest standard of care.

Addressing the complexities of geriatric dentistry through minimally invasive techniques necessitates a nuanced understanding of the physiological and pathological changes that occur with aging. The application of these techniques requires adaptation to the unique needs of older patients, whose oral health challenges are often compounded by systemic conditions, medication side effects, and decreased resilience to dental interventions.

One prominent issue in geriatric dentistry is the management of xerostomia, or dry mouth, which is frequently caused by medications, systemic diseases, or natural aging processes. Xerostomia significantly increases the risk of dental caries, oral infections, and discomfort. Minimally invasive approaches to managing xerostomia include the use of salivary substitutes, stimulants, and fluoride treatments. Salivary substitutes help moisten the oral cavity and alleviate discomfort, while salivary stimulants, such as sugar-free chewing gum or lozenges, can encourage natural saliva production. Regular fluoride applications, either in the form of varnishes or gels, are vital for protecting the teeth from decay, particularly in areas where saliva flow is compromised.

In managing tooth wear, which is a common concern among the elderly due to attrition, abrasion, and erosion, minimally invasive techniques focus on both prevention and conservative restoration. Preventive strategies may include the application of remineralizing agents, such as calcium phosphate or fluoride, to strengthen the tooth enamel and reduce sensitivity. For existing wear, minimal intervention techniques like bonding and the use of resin-based composites can restore tooth structure without extensive preparation. These methods align with the minimally invasive philosophy by preserving as much of the original tooth as possible while addressing functional and aesthetic concerns.

The treatment of root caries, a condition prevalent among older adults due to gingival recession and exposure of the tooth roots, requires particular attention. Minimally invasive treatments for root caries involve the application of fluoride, sealants, and minimally invasive restorations. Fluoride applications help to remineralize the exposed root surfaces and inhibit further decay. Sealants can be used to cover vulnerable root areas and prevent caries development. When restorative treatment is necessary, techniques such as atraumatic restorative treatment (ART) or resin infiltration can be employed to repair the damaged root with minimal tooth structure removal.

Periodontal health is another crucial aspect of geriatric dental care. As individuals age, they are at increased risk of periodontal disease, which can lead to tooth mobility and loss if not properly managed. Minimally invasive periodontal treatments include scaling and root planing with adjunctive therapies such as antimicrobial agents or laser treatment. These methods aim to remove plaque and calculus from the tooth surfaces and periodontal pockets with minimal discomfort and disruption. The use of lasers, for example, allows for precise tissue removal and bacterial decontamination, often resulting in quicker healing and reduced postoperative discomfort.

Moreover, the integration of technology into geriatric dental practice enhances the ability to provide minimally invasive care. The use of digital impressions, for instance, reduces the need for conventional, often uncomfortable, impression materials and provides more accurate and quicker results. This technology facilitates the creation of well-fitting restorations and prosthetics with minimal discomfort to the patient. Similarly, advanced imaging technologies, such as cone beam computed tomography (CBCT), provide detailed views of dental structures, aiding in precise diagnosis and treatment planning while reducing the need for invasive exploratory procedures.

Patient comfort remains a central concern in geriatric dentistry, particularly for those with diminished pain tolerance or complex medical histories. Minimally invasive techniques are designed to reduce discomfort and improve the overall patient experience. This includes the use of gentle, non-invasive diagnostic tools, and the application of local anesthesia or sedation as necessary to manage anxiety and pain. For patients with cognitive impairments or mobility issues, tailored approaches that involve clear communication, additional support, and accommodating physical needs are essential for ensuring a positive treatment experience.

Furthermore, the role of preventive care cannot be overstated in geriatric dentistry. Regular check-ups, tailored oral hygiene instructions, and proactive management of systemic conditions all contribute to the success of minimally invasive treatments. Preventive care strategies help in early detection of issues, thus enabling timely and conservative interventions. For example, patients with diabetes or cardiovascular disease benefit from personalized care plans that address both their systemic and oral health needs, promoting overall well-being and reducing the risk of dental complications.

In summary, the application of minimally invasive techniques in geriatric dentistry addresses the unique challenges faced by older adults, emphasizing a conservative approach to treatment that prioritizes patient comfort and preserves natural tooth structure. By integrating advanced technologies, preventive care, and tailored treatment strategies, dental professionals can effectively manage age-related dental issues and improve the overall oral health outcomes for their elderly patients. As the population continues to age, the evolution of minimally invasive techniques will remain essential in providing high-quality, patient-centered care that meets the diverse needs of geriatric patients.

In addition to addressing the direct dental issues faced by geriatric patients, minimally invasive techniques also involve a comprehensive approach to managing the broader health and functional aspects of aging. This holistic view is essential for optimizing patient outcomes and ensuring that interventions are not only effective but also aligned with the overall health and quality of life of older adults.

One key area of focus is the management of complex dental restorations, such as dentures or implants, in the elderly. For many older patients, traditional dentures may become uncomfortable or ill-fitting over time. Minimally invasive approaches to denture adjustments involve the use of modern materials and techniques to enhance comfort and function. For instance, the use of flexible denture materials can provide a more natural fit and greater comfort, while precision attachment systems can improve denture stability and retention. Similarly, implant-supported dentures offer a more secure and functional alternative to traditional removable dentures, with the minimally invasive placement of implants being guided by advanced imaging and computer-assisted techniques.

Another consideration in geriatric dentistry is the management of oral cancer and pre-cancerous lesions. Older adults are at a higher risk for oral cancer, and early detection is crucial for effective treatment. Minimally invasive diagnostic techniques, such as fluorescence imaging or brush biopsies, allow for the early identification of suspicious lesions with minimal discomfort to the patient. These techniques enable timely intervention, potentially reducing the need for more invasive surgical procedures and improving the overall prognosis for patients.

The integration of preventive care strategies is also vital for maintaining oral health in geriatric patients. Preventive care extends beyond routine cleanings and examinations to include tailored recommendations for oral hygiene practices and dietary modifications. For instance, patients with limited dexterity may benefit from the use of electric toothbrushes or other adaptive oral hygiene aids. Dietary counseling can address issues such as acid erosion or the impact of high sugar intake on oral health, helping to mitigate risks associated with aging-related changes in diet or saliva production.

Collaborative care is another essential component in managing geriatric patients. This involves working closely with other healthcare providers to address the complex interplay between oral health and overall health conditions. For example, patients with systemic diseases such as diabetes or cardiovascular conditions require coordinated care that integrates dental treatment with their broader medical management. Communication between dental professionals and primary care providers ensures that treatment plans are comprehensive and that any modifications in medication or health status are considered in the context of dental care.

The role of patient education cannot be understated in the context of geriatric dentistry. Educating patients and their caregivers about the importance of maintaining oral health, recognizing signs of dental issues, and understanding treatment options is crucial for effective self-management and adherence to care plans. This education should be tailored to the specific needs of older adults, considering factors such as cognitive impairments or sensory limitations. Providing clear, understandable information and engaging patients in their care fosters a sense of empowerment and can lead to better health outcomes.

In the realm of minimally invasive techniques, the use of digital technologies and telehealth has opened new avenues for improving care for elderly patients. Digital tools such as intraoral cameras and electronic health records facilitate more precise diagnostics and treatment planning, while telehealth services allow for remote consultations and follow-ups. These technologies can be particularly beneficial for elderly patients who may have difficulty accessing traditional in-person appointments due to mobility issues or transportation challenges.

Furthermore, the implementation of a patient-centered approach in minimally invasive geriatric dentistry emphasizes respect for the individual's preferences, values, and overall well-being. This approach involves engaging patients in discussions about their treatment goals, addressing their concerns and fears, and tailoring interventions to align with their lifestyle and health priorities. By prioritizing patient comfort and autonomy, dental professionals can enhance the overall experience and satisfaction of older patients, contributing to more successful and sustainable outcomes.

In conclusion, the application of minimally invasive techniques in geriatric dentistry addresses the multifaceted needs of older adults by focusing on conservative, effective, and patient-centered care. These techniques are designed to improve comfort, preserve natural tooth structure, and manage age-related dental issues while integrating with broader health considerations. As the population of older adults continues to grow, the evolution of minimally invasive techniques will play a crucial role in advancing geriatric dental care, ensuring that treatments are both effective and respectful of the unique needs of this diverse and aging demographic.

CHAPTER 37: THE ROLE OF DIGITAL TOOLS IN MINIMALLY INVASIVE DENTISTRY

The advent of digital tools and technologies has significantly transformed the landscape of minimally invasive dentistry. These advancements enhance the precision, efficiency, and outcomes of dental procedures by integrating sophisticated digital solutions into everyday practice. The convergence of digital imaging, computer-aided design and manufacturing (CAD/CAM) systems, and other innovative tools represents a pivotal shift towards more accurate and patient-centered dental care.

Digital imaging is a cornerstone of modern minimally invasive dentistry. Techniques such as digital radiography and intraoral cameras have revolutionized diagnostic accuracy and treatment planning. Digital radiography, for example, offers superior image quality with reduced radiation exposure compared to traditional film-based methods. This technology allows for immediate image acquisition and evaluation, facilitating quicker diagnosis and more effective treatment planning. The ability to enhance, magnify, and adjust digital images also aids in identifying subtle issues that may not be visible with conventional methods.

Intraoral cameras further contribute to the diagnostic process by providing detailed, real-time images of the oral cavity. These cameras capture high-resolution images of teeth, gums, and other oral structures, allowing for comprehensive visual assessments. The integration of these images into digital patient records supports precise documentation and enables enhanced communication with patients. Visual evidence of dental conditions can be used to explain treatment options and procedures, thereby improving patient understanding and engagement.

Computer-aided design and manufacturing (CAD/CAM) systems represent another significant advancement in minimally invasive dentistry. CAD/CAM technology enables the precise design and fabrication of dental restorations, such as crowns, veneers, and inlays, directly from digital impressions. This process eliminates the need for traditional impressions, which can be uncomfortable for patients and prone to inaccuracies. Digital impressions, obtained through intraoral scanners, provide a more comfortable experience and yield highly accurate data for restoration design.

The CAD portion of the system involves creating detailed digital models of the teeth and surrounding structures. Advanced software allows dental professionals to design restorations with exceptional precision, tailoring them to the individual patient's anatomy. The CAM component then utilizes this digital design to mill or fabricate the restoration from a block of material, such as ceramic or composite. This streamlined process reduces the time required for restoration fabrication and allows for same-day treatments, enhancing patient convenience and satisfaction.

Additionally, the role of digital tools extends to the realm of surgical planning and execution. Technologies such as cone beam computed tomography (CBCT) offer three-dimensional imaging that provides detailed views of bone structure and tooth alignment. This advanced imaging capability is particularly valuable in planning minimally invasive surgical procedures, such as implant placements. By visualizing the anatomical structures in three dimensions, dental professionals can make informed decisions regarding implant positioning, reducing the risk of complications and improving overall outcomes.

Guided surgery systems, which often integrate with CBCT imaging, further enhance the precision of minimally invasive procedures. These systems use computer-generated surgical guides to assist in the accurate placement of implants or other devices. The guides are based on digital treatment plans and are designed to fit precisely in the patient's mouth, ensuring that the surgical procedure is performed with high accuracy. This approach minimizes the need for flap surgeries and reduces post-operative discomfort, contributing to a faster recovery and improved patient experience.

The integration of digital tools also supports better workflow management and documentation. Electronic health records (EHR) and practice management software facilitate the organization of patient information, treatment plans, and clinical notes. These systems enable seamless data sharing between different components of the practice, such as diagnostic imaging, treatment planning, and patient communication. The accessibility of digital records improves coordination among dental professionals and enhances the continuity of care.

Moreover, digital tools play a crucial role in patient education and engagement. The use of digital simulations and visual aids helps patients visualize the potential outcomes of various treatment options. For instance, digital smile design software allows patients to see a preview of their post-treatment appearance, which can be a powerful motivator for proceeding with recommended procedures. Enhanced patient engagement through these tools fosters a better understanding of treatment options and promotes informed decision-making.

The integration of digital technologies in minimally invasive dentistry is not without its challenges. The initial cost of acquiring and maintaining advanced digital equipment can be substantial, and there is a learning curve associated with mastering these technologies. However, the benefits they offer in terms of improved precision, efficiency, and patient satisfaction often outweigh these considerations. As technology continues to advance, it is expected that digital tools will become increasingly accessible and integral to dental practice.

In summary, digital tools have become essential in advancing minimally invasive dentistry, offering improvements in diagnostic accuracy, treatment planning, and patient care. The integration of digital imaging, CAD/CAM systems, and guided surgery technologies enhances the precision and efficiency of dental procedures while providing a more comfortable experience for patients. As these technologies evolve, they will continue to play a pivotal role in shaping the future of minimally invasive dentistry, driving further innovations and enhancing overall oral health outcomes.

The transformative impact of digital tools on minimally invasive dentistry extends beyond the confines of individual procedures, influencing the broader scope of dental practice management and patient interaction. One of the notable advancements is the integration of digital tools into patient communication and education, a critical element in ensuring successful treatment outcomes.

Digital communication platforms allow for the seamless sharing of information between dental professionals and patients. Through digital portals, patients can access their treatment plans, review educational materials, and track their progress in real time. This transparency fosters a better understanding of treatment goals and procedures, which can significantly influence patient satisfaction and adherence to care recommendations. For instance, patients who are well-informed about their procedures are more likely to have realistic expectations and engage positively in their treatment.

Another dimension of digital innovation in minimally invasive dentistry is the development of virtual and augmented reality tools. These technologies provide immersive experiences that enhance patient understanding of complex procedures. Virtual reality can simulate various dental scenarios, allowing patients to visualize the outcomes of different treatment options. Augmented reality, on the other hand, can overlay digital information onto the physical environment, offering real-time guidance during treatments. These technologies not only improve patient education but also aid clinicians in performing procedures with greater precision and confidence.

The role of digital tools also extends to the realm of preventive care and monitoring. Digital platforms and mobile applications are increasingly being used to support oral health maintenance outside the clinical setting. For example, mobile apps that track oral hygiene practices can provide patients with reminders and feedback on their brushing and flossing routines. Some apps even incorporate AI-driven analysis to offer personalized recommendations based on user data. This continuous engagement helps reinforce the principles of preventive care and encourages patients to maintain optimal oral health practices.

Moreover, the integration of digital tools facilitates more efficient and effective management of dental practices. Advanced practice management software streamlines administrative tasks such as scheduling, billing, and patient record management. These systems offer comprehensive solutions that enhance operational efficiency and reduce the administrative burden on dental professionals. By automating routine tasks and providing detailed analytics, these tools allow practitioners to focus more on clinical care and less on paperwork.

One significant area where digital tools have made an impact is in the realm of evidence-based practice. The integration of digital databases and research platforms enables dental professionals to access the latest clinical guidelines and research findings with ease. This access to up-to-date information supports the implementation of evidence-based treatment protocols and fosters continuous professional development. By staying informed about the latest advancements and best practices, practitioners can ensure that their minimally invasive techniques are grounded in current scientific evidence.

Additionally, digital tools enhance the ability to conduct and participate in collaborative research. Digital platforms facilitate data sharing and collaboration among researchers, enabling the pooling of resources and knowledge. Collaborative research projects can lead to the development of new techniques and innovations in minimally invasive dentistry, further advancing the field. The ability to analyze large datasets and perform complex statistical analyses using digital tools also contributes to the advancement of evidence-based practices.

Despite the many advantages offered by digital tools, it is important to acknowledge the challenges associated with their integration into dental practice. The initial investment in digital equipment and software can be substantial, and the ongoing maintenance costs must be considered. Additionally, there is a need for training and education to ensure that dental professionals are proficient in using these technologies.

As with any technological advancement, there is also the potential for issues related to data security and privacy that must be addressed to protect patient information.

Looking ahead, the future of digital tools in minimally invasive dentistry holds exciting possibilities. The continued evolution of artificial intelligence (AI) and machine learning is likely to bring further advancements in diagnostic accuracy and treatment planning. AI algorithms can analyze vast amounts of data to identify patterns and make predictions, potentially leading to earlier detection of dental conditions and more personalized treatment approaches. The integration of AI into digital imaging and treatment planning tools could revolutionize the way minimally invasive procedures are performed.

In conclusion, digital tools play a crucial role in enhancing minimally invasive dentistry by improving precision, efficiency, and patient outcomes. The integration of advanced imaging, CAD/CAM systems, and digital communication platforms has transformed various aspects of dental practice, from diagnosis and treatment planning to patient education and practice management. While challenges remain, the ongoing advancements in digital technology promise to further elevate the standards of minimally invasive care, ultimately contributing to better oral health and improved patient experiences.

The deployment of digital tools in minimally invasive dentistry extends to the realms of patient assessment and treatment planning, where precision and customization are paramount. One notable advancement in this area is the use of digital imaging techniques, which have fundamentally transformed the approach to diagnostics and treatment planning. Traditional imaging methods, while useful, often lacked the level of detail and accuracy required for the optimal planning of minimally invasive procedures. Digital imaging technologies, such as cone beam computed tomography (CBCT) and intraoral cameras, address these limitations by providing high-resolution images that facilitate more accurate diagnoses and treatment planning.

CBCT, in particular, offers a three-dimensional view of the dental structures, allowing clinicians to visualize the spatial relationships between teeth, bone, and surrounding tissues. This enhanced visualization is crucial for planning procedures such as dental implants, where precise placement is essential for long-term success. The ability to assess bone density, volume, and the proximity of critical anatomical structures in three dimensions enables practitioners to plan treatments with greater accuracy and reduce the risk of complications. Furthermore, CBCT images can be integrated with digital impression data to create comprehensive treatment plans that consider all relevant factors, improving the overall efficacy of minimally invasive interventions.

Intraoral cameras provide another layer of detail by capturing close-up images of the oral cavity, which can be used to document and monitor changes over time. These images enhance the clinician's ability to identify early signs of dental issues, such as carious lesions or gum disease, at a stage when minimally invasive treatments are most effective. Additionally, intraoral cameras facilitate patient education by allowing patients to see real-time images of their oral health, thereby fostering a better understanding of their condition and the proposed treatment plan.

The integration of Computer-Aided Design and Computer-Aided Manufacturing (CAD/CAM) systems represents another significant advancement in minimally invasive dentistry. CAD/CAM technology enables the digital design and fabrication of dental restorations, such as crowns, veneers, and inlays, with remarkable precision. The process begins with the acquisition of a digital impression, which is then used to create a virtual model of the patient's dentition. This model allows for the design of restorations that are tailored to the individual's unique anatomical and functional requirements.

Once the design is complete, CAD/CAM systems facilitate the milling or 3D printing of the restoration from high-quality materials. This streamlined process reduces the need for multiple patient visits and the reliance on traditional, often less precise, impression techniques. The result is a restoration that fits with greater accuracy, minimizes the need for adjustments, and enhances the overall patient experience. Moreover, the use of CAD/CAM technology supports minimally invasive approaches by enabling the design and fabrication of restorations that preserve more of the natural tooth structure compared to conventional methods.

Digital tools also play a critical role in enhancing procedural efficiency and outcomes through real-time feedback and guidance. Technologies such as digital guided surgery systems provide navigational support during procedures, ensuring that treatments are performed with the highest degree of accuracy. For instance, during implant placement, guided surgery systems use preoperative imaging data to create a virtual surgical guide that directs the precise placement of implants. This approach not only improves the accuracy of the procedure but also reduces the risk of complications and shortens recovery times.

Furthermore, digital tools contribute to improved outcomes by facilitating the implementation of evidence-based practices. Access to digital libraries and databases allows dental practitioners to stay informed about the latest research and clinical guidelines. This continuous access to up-to-date information supports the integration of evidence-based techniques into daily practice, enhancing the effectiveness of minimally invasive treatments.

As digital tools continue to evolve, their integration into minimally invasive dentistry will likely lead to further advancements. Emerging technologies, such as artificial intelligence and machine learning, hold the potential to revolutionize diagnostic accuracy and treatment planning. AI algorithms can analyze vast amounts of data to identify patterns and predict outcomes, offering new insights that can inform treatment decisions. For example, AI-driven diagnostic tools may assist in the early detection of dental conditions by analyzing digital images and identifying subtle changes that may indicate the onset of disease.

Despite the many benefits of digital tools, it is important to address the challenges associated with their use. The rapid pace of technological advancement requires ongoing education and training for dental professionals to remain proficient in utilizing these tools. Additionally, the initial investment and maintenance costs of digital equipment can be significant, necessitating careful consideration and planning. Ensuring data security and privacy also remains a priority, as the protection of patient information is paramount in maintaining trust and compliance with regulations.

In summary, the role of digital tools in minimally invasive dentistry is pivotal in advancing the field through improved precision, efficiency, and patient outcomes. Digital imaging, CAD/CAM systems, and real-time feedback technologies collectively enhance the diagnostic and treatment capabilities of dental practitioners. As technology continues to advance, the integration of digital tools will likely further refine minimally invasive practices, offering even greater benefits to both patients and practitioners. The continued evolution of digital technologies promises to drive innovation in dental care, ultimately contributing to more effective and patient-centered minimally invasive treatments.

CHAPTER 38: MINIMALLY INVASIVE APPROACHES TO MANAGING DENTAL HYPERSENSITIVITY

Dental hypersensitivity, characterized by sharp pain or discomfort in response to certain stimuli, presents a significant challenge in clinical practice. Traditionally, the management of this condition often involved more invasive procedures, potentially compromising tooth structure. However, advancements in minimally invasive dentistry offer promising alternatives that emphasize preservation of natural tooth structure while effectively addressing hypersensitivity.

To approach dental hypersensitivity with minimally invasive techniques, one must first understand the underlying causes of the condition. Hypersensitivity typically arises from the exposure of dentin, the layer of tooth structure beneath the enamel, which contains microscopic tubules that connect to the nerve endings within the tooth. Various factors such as enamel erosion, gum recession, and aggressive brushing can contribute to this exposure. Effective management thus begins with a comprehensive diagnostic assessment to identify the specific etiology of the hypersensitivity.

A key component in the minimally invasive management of hypersensitivity is the use of conservative treatment options. These treatments aim to protect and repair the exposed dentin while preserving as much of the tooth's natural structure as possible. One of the first-line conservative treatments involves the application of desensitizing agents. These agents, which include fluoride varnishes and calcium phosphates, work by occluding the dentinal tubules or enhancing the remineralization of enamel and dentin. The application of fluoride varnishes, for example, can help to form a protective layer over the exposed dentin, reducing the transmission of stimuli to the nerves. Calcium phosphate compounds, on the other hand, assist in restoring lost minerals to the tooth structure, promoting repair and reducing sensitivity.

Another conservative approach involves the use of bonding agents or sealants to cover exposed dentin. These materials, typically applied as a thin layer, create a barrier that blocks the tubules and insulates the dentin from external stimuli. The application process is minimally invasive, involving careful cleaning of the tooth surface and the application of a bonding resin that hardens to form a protective layer. This method not only alleviates sensitivity but also helps in preserving the integrity of the tooth structure.

For patients with hypersensitivity related to gum recession, periodontal therapies can be particularly effective. Techniques such as scaling and root planing help to address the underlying gum disease that may be contributing to the recession. In cases where recession has already occurred, minimally invasive surgical options, such as connective tissue grafts or collagen-based materials, can be employed to cover exposed roots and improve gum health. These procedures are designed to be as conservative as possible, focusing on tissue regeneration and protection rather than extensive surgical intervention.

In addition to these direct treatments, it is essential to incorporate preventive strategies into the management plan. Educating patients about proper oral hygiene practices can significantly reduce the risk of hypersensitivity. Emphasizing the importance of using a soft-bristled toothbrush and avoiding excessive brushing pressure can help prevent further enamel erosion and gum recession. Additionally, recommending toothpaste formulated for sensitive teeth can offer ongoing relief by blocking the dentinal tubules and strengthening the enamel.

Diagnostic approaches in the management of dental hypersensitivity also benefit from minimally invasive techniques. Modern diagnostic tools, such as digital imaging and transillumination, allow for precise assessment of tooth structure and identification of areas susceptible to hypersensitivity. Digital radiographs provide detailed views of tooth and bone structures, helping to detect underlying issues that may be contributing to sensitivity. Transillumination uses light to examine the translucency of tooth structure, revealing areas of potential damage or weakness. These non-invasive diagnostic methods facilitate accurate diagnosis and tailored treatment planning without the need for invasive procedures.

Addressing dental hypersensitivity through minimally invasive methods not only alleviates discomfort but also contributes to the long-term health and preservation of dental structures. By focusing on conservative treatments and preventive measures, practitioners can effectively manage hypersensitivity while minimizing the impact on tooth structure. This approach aligns with the principles of minimally invasive dentistry, which prioritize the preservation of natural tooth material and the application of the least invasive techniques necessary to achieve therapeutic goals.

In summary, the management of dental hypersensitivity through minimally invasive approaches offers significant benefits in terms of preserving tooth structure and improving patient comfort. Conservative treatments such as desensitizing agents, bonding agents, and preventive strategies play a crucial role in addressing the underlying causes of hypersensitivity while maintaining the integrity of the tooth. The use of advanced diagnostic tools further enhances the ability to accurately identify and treat hypersensitivity in a minimally invasive manner. As the field of minimally invasive dentistry continues to evolve, ongoing research and development in these areas promise to enhance the effectiveness and comfort of hypersensitivity management, contributing to improved oral health outcomes and patient satisfaction.

In the management of dental hypersensitivity, understanding patient-specific factors and customizing treatment strategies is essential for effective outcomes. Minimally invasive approaches focus not only on alleviating symptoms but also on addressing the root causes of hypersensitivity while preserving the integrity of the dental structure.

One innovative minimally invasive technique involves the use of laser therapy. Lasers can be employed to treat hypersensitivity by selectively targeting and sealing dentinal tubules, thereby reducing their sensitivity to external stimuli. The precision of laser technology allows for targeted treatment with minimal impact on surrounding tissues. This approach can be particularly beneficial for patients with localized sensitivity, providing quick relief while maintaining tooth structure. Additionally, laser therapy may promote the formation of a protective layer on the dentin, further reducing sensitivity and enhancing overall treatment efficacy.

Another advanced technique is the application of bioactive glass materials. Bioactive glasses are compounds that can bond to dental hard tissues and release beneficial ions, such as calcium and phosphate, which promote remineralization and strengthen the tooth structure. When applied to areas of hypersensitivity, bioactive glass materials form a protective layer over exposed dentin, helping to occlude tubules and reduce discomfort. The application of these materials is minimally invasive, involving the careful placement of the glass on the affected area, and can be integrated into a comprehensive treatment plan that includes other conservative measures.

Minimally invasive management of dental hypersensitivity also includes the consideration of patient-specific lifestyle factors and habits. For instance, dietary habits that contribute to enamel erosion, such as high consumption of acidic foods and beverages, should be addressed. Providing patients with dietary counseling and recommending modifications can help prevent further damage and reduce sensitivity. Additionally, habits such as bruxism, or teeth grinding, may exacerbate hypersensitivity by causing mechanical wear on tooth surfaces. In such cases, the use of occlusal splints or night guards can protect the teeth from excessive wear and alleviate associated sensitivity.

The integration of patient education into the management strategy is critical. Educating patients about the nature of their condition, the causes of hypersensitivity, and the available treatment options empowers them to make informed decisions about their care. Clear communication regarding the expected outcomes of various treatments and the importance of adhering to recommended preventive measures can significantly enhance the effectiveness of minimally invasive approaches. Providing patients with guidance on proper oral hygiene practices, such as the use of fluoride toothpaste and soft-bristled brushes, can help maintain the health of their teeth and reduce the risk of developing sensitivity in the future.

In addition to individual treatment strategies, a multidisciplinary approach can enhance the management of hypersensitivity. Collaboration with dental hygienists, periodontists, and other specialists may be necessary to address underlying conditions that contribute to hypersensitivity. For example, if gum recession is a contributing factor, periodontal treatments to address gum health may be required in conjunction with other conservative measures. Similarly, coordination with a dental technician for custom-made dental appliances can offer additional support and protection for patients experiencing severe sensitivity.

Finally, ongoing evaluation and follow-up are crucial components of a minimally invasive management plan. Regular monitoring of patient progress allows for adjustments to the treatment approach based on the effectiveness and patient feedback. Follow-up appointments provide an opportunity to assess the success of the initial interventions, address any new concerns, and reinforce preventive strategies. This iterative process ensures that the management plan remains responsive to the patient's needs and continues to deliver optimal outcomes over time.

In summary, the minimally invasive management of dental hypersensitivity involves a combination of advanced techniques, conservative treatments, and personalized care. By focusing on precision and preservation, these approaches address the symptoms of hypersensitivity while maintaining the health and integrity of the tooth structure. The use of technologies such as laser therapy and bioactive glasses, combined with lifestyle modifications and patient education, offers a comprehensive strategy for managing hypersensitivity effectively. Collaboration with dental professionals and ongoing evaluation further enhance the success of minimally invasive treatments, ultimately contributing to improved patient comfort and satisfaction.

The management of dental hypersensitivity through minimally invasive techniques represents a crucial advancement in maintaining oral health and patient comfort. Central to these approaches is a careful balance between alleviating symptoms and preserving the natural structure of the teeth. Understanding how to implement these methods effectively requires a nuanced approach to both diagnosis and treatment, ensuring that interventions are both targeted and gentle.

One key aspect of managing dental hypersensitivity is the accurate diagnosis of its underlying causes. Hypersensitivity can result from a variety of factors including enamel erosion, dentin exposure, and gingival recession. Each of these conditions requires a tailored approach to treatment. For instance, enamel erosion caused by acidic foods or beverages can be managed through dietary counseling and the application of remineralizing agents. Fluoride varnishes or calcium phosphate products can help to strengthen the remaining enamel and protect against further erosion. This strategy not only addresses the symptoms but also works to prevent the progression of enamel loss, providing a holistic approach to managing hypersensitivity.

Dentin exposure, which occurs when the protective enamel is worn away or when gums recede, can be treated with materials that occlude dentinal tubules and reduce sensitivity. The application of desensitizing agents, such as potassium nitrate or fluoride, can help to block the pathways through which stimuli reach the nerve endings in the dentin. These agents are applied directly to the affected areas and work by interrupting the transmission of nerve impulses, thereby reducing discomfort. The choice of agent and application technique must be carefully considered based on the patient's specific condition and response to previous treatments.

Gingival recession, another common cause of hypersensitivity, requires a different set of interventions. Techniques such as guided tissue regeneration or soft tissue grafts can be employed to address the underlying periodontal issues. Minimally invasive surgical techniques, including the use of collagen membranes and connective tissue grafts, allow for the restoration of gingival tissue with minimal discomfort and faster recovery compared to more invasive procedures. Additionally, the use of non-surgical periodontal therapy, such as scaling and root planing, can help manage gingival inflammation and recession while preserving natural tissue.

In addition to these specific treatments, the use of advanced technologies and diagnostic tools enhances the effectiveness of minimally invasive approaches. Digital imaging techniques, such as intraoral cameras and cone-beam computed tomography (CBCT), provide detailed views of the tooth structure and surrounding tissues. These tools enable precise diagnosis of hypersensitivity and allow for the planning of targeted treatments. The ability to visualize and assess the extent of enamel loss, dentin exposure, or gingival recession in detail supports more accurate treatment planning and better outcomes.

Moreover, patient education plays a critical role in the successful management of dental hypersensitivity. Educating patients about the causes of their sensitivity, the importance of adhering to preventive measures, and the benefits of recommended treatments empowers them to take an active role in their oral health. Instruction on proper brushing techniques, the use of desensitizing toothpaste, and dietary modifications can significantly impact the management of hypersensitivity. By equipping patients with knowledge and practical strategies, dental professionals can enhance treatment efficacy and improve overall patient satisfaction.

Finally, ongoing follow-up and monitoring are essential components of a minimally invasive management plan. Regular check-ups allow for the assessment of treatment effectiveness, the identification of any new issues, and the adjustment of strategies as needed. This iterative process ensures that interventions remain effective over time and that any emerging symptoms are addressed promptly. Follow-up appointments also provide an opportunity to reinforce patient education, evaluate adherence to recommended practices, and make any necessary adjustments to the treatment plan.

In summary, the management of dental hypersensitivity using minimally invasive techniques encompasses a range of strategies designed to alleviate symptoms while preserving tooth structure. From conservative treatments like fluoride applications and bioactive glass to advanced diagnostic tools and patient education, these approaches focus on providing effective relief with minimal disruption to the natural anatomy of the teeth. By combining precise diagnosis, targeted treatment, and ongoing patient engagement, dental professionals can successfully manage hypersensitivity and enhance patient comfort and satisfaction.

CHAPTER 39: PATIENT EDUCATION AND ENGAGEMENT IN MINIMALLY INVASIVE DENTISTRY

Effective patient education and engagement are pivotal in the practice of minimally invasive dentistry, where the emphasis is placed on preserving natural tooth structure and using conservative treatment methods. The success of these techniques largely hinges on how well patients understand their treatment options, the benefits of these options, and how they can participate in their own oral health management.

Central to patient education is the clear and comprehensive communication of what minimally invasive dentistry entails. Patients must be informed about the philosophy behind these techniques, which prioritize the preservation of healthy tooth structure while addressing dental issues with the least possible intervention. This approach not only aims to reduce the physical impact of treatments but also seeks to enhance long-term oral health and patient satisfaction. A fundamental aspect of this communication is ensuring that patients grasp the rationale behind choosing minimally invasive methods over more traditional, invasive options. By elucidating the principles of conservative care, dental professionals can help patients appreciate the value of preserving natural dentition and avoiding unnecessary procedures.

To facilitate effective patient education, it is crucial to use various tools and methods that accommodate different learning styles and preferences. Visual aids such as diagrams, videos, and interactive models can be particularly useful in illustrating complex concepts related to minimally invasive techniques. For instance, digital simulations or animated videos can vividly demonstrate how procedures are performed and how they benefit the patient. Such visual tools help demystify treatments and provide a clearer understanding of the procedures, which can alleviate patient anxiety and foster a sense of trust in the dental team.

Moreover, engaging patients in their care decisions is essential for fostering a collaborative approach to oral health. This involves actively involving patients in discussions about their treatment options, including the benefits and potential drawbacks of each approach. When patients are given a voice in their care, they are more likely to be committed to following through with the recommended treatments. Shared decision-making models, where patients and practitioners work together to choose the best course of action, can lead to improved adherence to treatment plans and better overall outcomes. This collaborative approach not only empowers patients but also helps build a therapeutic alliance between the patient and the dental team.

An important component of patient engagement is the development of a personalized care plan that addresses the unique needs and preferences of each individual. Personalized care plans should consider factors such as the patient's oral health history, specific dental concerns, and personal goals for treatment. By tailoring care plans to individual needs, dental professionals can ensure that treatments are aligned with the patient's expectations and that they address their specific issues effectively. This individualized approach also allows for the incorporation of patient feedback, which can further enhance their engagement and satisfaction with the care they receive.

In addition to providing information about specific treatments, dental professionals should also focus on educating patients about preventive measures and self-care practices that support oral health. This includes guidance on proper brushing and flossing techniques, dietary recommendations, and the importance of regular dental check-ups. Preventive education is a cornerstone of minimally invasive dentistry, as it helps patients understand how to maintain their oral health proactively and reduce the need for more invasive interventions in the future. By emphasizing the importance of routine care and preventive practices, dental professionals can help patients take an active role in managing their oral health.

Effective patient engagement also involves addressing and managing any concerns or misconceptions that patients may have about minimally invasive procedures. Providing clear and empathetic responses to questions about the efficacy, safety, and potential outcomes of treatments can help alleviate concerns and build confidence in the chosen approach. Additionally, creating an open and supportive environment where patients feel comfortable expressing their fears or uncertainties can lead to more honest discussions and better-informed decisions.

Finally, follow-up and ongoing communication play a critical role in maintaining patient engagement. Regular check-ins, both during and after treatment, allow for the monitoring of progress, the addressing of any issues that arise, and the reinforcement of preventive care practices. Follow-up appointments also provide an opportunity to discuss any further questions or concerns that patients may have, thereby continuing the education process and ensuring that patients remain informed and engaged in their care.

In summary, patient education and engagement are integral to the successful implementation of minimally invasive dentistry. By employing clear communication, using various educational tools, involving patients in decision-making, and focusing on preventive care, dental professionals can enhance patient understanding and satisfaction. This proactive approach not only improves the effectiveness of minimally invasive treatments but also fosters a collaborative and supportive relationship between patients and their dental care providers.

When it comes to patient education and engagement in minimally invasive dentistry, a strategic approach is essential to ensure that patients are well-informed and actively involved in their oral health care. One of the critical aspects of this process is the establishment of a clear and consistent communication framework. This begins with the initial consultation, where the goals and benefits of minimally invasive techniques should be thoroughly explained. By laying a strong foundation of understanding from the outset, dental professionals can help patients make informed decisions about their treatment options.

A key component of effective patient education is the use of understandable and relatable language. Avoiding overly technical jargon and instead using terms that patients can easily grasp is crucial. For instance, rather than discussing the specifics of enamel remineralization in technical terms, explaining it as a way to strengthen the tooth and prevent decay can be more accessible. This approach helps demystify the procedures and makes the information more relatable, thereby enhancing patient comprehension.

In addition to verbal explanations, incorporating visual

aids can significantly enhance patient understanding. High-quality digital images, diagrams, and animations can provide a clear depiction of what to expect before, during, and after a procedure. These tools help bridge the gap between complex dental concepts and patient understanding. For instance, before showing a patient a specific procedure, using a visual aid to illustrate the problem and the minimally invasive solution can make the treatment plan more concrete and less intimidating.

Educational brochures and pamphlets can also be valuable resources for reinforcing information provided during consultations. These materials allow patients to review the details of their treatment at their own pace, which can be particularly helpful in reducing anxiety and ensuring that they fully grasp the implications of their choices. Brochures should be designed to be patient-friendly, with clear headings, simple language, and engaging visuals.

Another effective method for patient education is the use of digital platforms, such as practice websites and patient portals. These platforms can offer a wealth of information, including educational videos, FAQs, and interactive content that patients can access at their convenience. Incorporating a section on minimally invasive techniques, complete with patient testimonials and case studies, can help patients feel more connected to their treatment options and the positive outcomes associated with them.

Involving patients in their care decisions requires a collaborative approach that respects their preferences and values. This involves presenting all viable treatment options, including the pros and cons of each, and encouraging patients to voice their concerns and preferences. Providing a balanced view of the potential outcomes of each option helps patients feel empowered to make decisions that align with their personal health goals and lifestyle.

Shared decision-making tools can facilitate this process by providing structured ways for patients to weigh their options and make informed choices. For example, decision aids such as comparison charts and risk calculators can help patients understand how different treatments might impact their health and quality of life. These tools also foster a sense of involvement and ownership in the treatment process, which can lead to greater satisfaction with the care received.

Engaging patients also involves addressing their concerns and answering their questions thoroughly. A patient's apprehension about a procedure can often be alleviated through open dialogue and reassurance. It is important for dental professionals to actively listen to patients, validate their concerns, and provide clear and honest answers. This approach not only builds trust but also helps to reduce anxiety and resistance to treatment.

Furthermore, fostering a proactive approach to oral health involves emphasizing the importance of preventive care. Educating patients about how daily habits, such as proper brushing and flossing, can significantly impact their oral health helps reinforce the value of ongoing self-care. Providing personalized recommendations and demonstrating techniques during appointments can further support patients in adopting effective oral hygiene practices.

Implementing follow-up strategies is also crucial for maintaining patient engagement. Regular check-ins, whether through phone calls, emails, or subsequent appointments, offer opportunities to discuss progress, address any new concerns, and reinforce the importance of continued care. These interactions not only keep patients informed but also demonstrate a commitment to their long-term health and well-being.

In summary, effective patient education and engagement in

minimally invasive dentistry involve clear communication, the use of visual aids, and the application of educational resources both in-person and digitally. By actively involving patients in their care decisions and emphasizing the importance of preventive measures, dental professionals can foster a collaborative relationship that enhances patient satisfaction and improves treatment outcomes. This approach ensures that patients are not only well-informed but also motivated to participate actively in their oral health management, leading to better overall results and a more positive dental experience.

A crucial element in maintaining effective patient engagement is the ongoing education and support provided throughout the treatment process. Beyond initial consultations and educational materials, continuous patient education ensures that individuals remain informed and involved at every stage of their care. This ongoing dialogue is vital for reinforcing the importance of follow-up care and addressing any concerns or questions that arise as patients progress through their treatment plans.

To enhance patient understanding and adherence to minimally invasive treatments, dental practices can employ various tools and strategies. One approach involves the use of tailored patient education plans that outline specific instructions and recommendations based on each individual's unique needs. These plans can include customized oral hygiene routines, dietary guidelines, and reminders about the importance of regular check-ups. By personalizing these recommendations, dental professionals can help patients better understand how their daily habits directly impact their treatment outcomes and overall oral health.

Digital technology plays a significant role in supporting patient education and engagement. For instance, interactive apps and online platforms can offer patients personalized guidance on their oral health routines, track their progress, and provide instant access to educational content. These tools can also facilitate communication between patients and their dental care team, allowing for quick responses to questions or concerns. Incorporating reminders and alerts within these platforms can help patients adhere to treatment plans and preventive measures.

Another important aspect of patient education is addressing the psychological and emotional dimensions of dental care. Minimally invasive procedures, while generally less intimidating than more invasive options, can still cause anxiety for some patients. Providing reassurance through empathetic communication and supportive interactions helps to alleviate these concerns. Educating patients about the gentle nature of minimally invasive techniques and the minimal discomfort they may experience can contribute to a more positive perception of their treatment.

In addition to direct education and communication, dental practices can benefit from implementing patient feedback mechanisms. Soliciting feedback from patients about their experiences and the effectiveness of the educational materials provided allows for continuous improvement in patient engagement strategies. Practices can use surveys, comment cards, or digital feedback tools to gather insights and make necessary adjustments to their approach. This iterative process ensures that patient education remains relevant and effective, addressing any gaps or issues that may arise.

Patient education is also enhanced through community outreach and public education initiatives. Dental practices can engage in activities such as hosting seminars, workshops, or webinars focused on oral health topics relevant to minimally invasive dentistry. These events not only provide valuable information to a broader audience but also establish the practice as a resource for oral health education. By fostering a culture of learning and awareness within the community, dental professionals can encourage proactive approaches to oral health care.

Collaboration with other healthcare providers can further support patient education and engagement. For instance, integrating dental care with broader health management plans, especially for patients with chronic conditions or complex health needs, ensures a comprehensive approach to their overall well-being. Coordinating with primary care physicians or specialists can provide patients with a more holistic view of how their dental health intersects with their overall health, reinforcing the importance of maintaining regular dental visits and adhering to recommended treatments.

Finally, it is essential for dental professionals to model and encourage self-care practices that align with the principles of minimally invasive dentistry. Demonstrating proper brushing and flossing techniques, discussing the benefits of fluoride use, and providing personalized advice on maintaining oral health are all integral to patient education. Encouraging patients to take an active role in their oral care, while providing the support and resources they need, fosters a sense of responsibility and empowerment.

In conclusion, effective patient education and engagement in minimally invasive dentistry are multifaceted processes that require clear communication, personalized care, and ongoing support. By leveraging a range of educational tools and strategies, including digital resources, tailored plans, and community outreach, dental professionals can enhance patient understanding and involvement in their care. Addressing the psychological aspects of dental treatment, soliciting patient feedback, and collaborating with other healthcare providers further contribute to a comprehensive approach to patient engagement. Ultimately, these efforts lead to improved patient satisfaction, better treatment outcomes, and a more proactive approach to oral health.

CHAPTER 40: INNOVATIONS IN BIOMATERIALS FOR MINIMALLY INVASIVE DENTISTRY

In the evolving field of minimally invasive dentistry, the role of advanced biomaterials is pivotal. These materials not only facilitate the conservative approach inherent to minimally invasive techniques but also significantly impact the durability, functionality, and aesthetic outcomes of dental restorations. As dental technology progresses, so too does the sophistication of biomaterials, which are continually refined to meet the demands of modern dental practice.

Composite resins represent one of the most dynamic areas of innovation within dental biomaterials. Recent developments have led to composites that offer improved mechanical properties, better wear resistance, and enhanced aesthetic qualities. Advances in nanotechnology have been particularly influential in this domain, leading to the creation of nanofilled composites. These materials incorporate nanoparticles that improve the strength and polishability of the resin, resulting in restorations that are more resistant to staining and wear. The enhanced mechanical properties of these composites allow for the successful treatment of a wider range of clinical situations with minimally invasive techniques, including the restoration of large cavities and the repair of fractured teeth.

The evolution of dental ceramics has also contributed significantly to minimally invasive dentistry. Traditional ceramics, while durable, often required substantial tooth reduction to accommodate their thickness. However, recent innovations in ceramic materials, such as high-strength zirconia and lithium disilicate, have enabled the development of ultra-thin veneers and inlays that preserve more of the natural tooth structure. These newer ceramics are not only stronger and more resistant to chipping but also offer superior aesthetics due to their translucency, which closely mimics the appearance of natural teeth. This advancement is particularly beneficial in cosmetic procedures, where maintaining a natural appearance is paramount.

Another notable advancement in biomaterials is the development of bioactive materials, which interact positively with biological tissues. Bioactive glass and certain types of calcium silicate-based materials are examples of this innovation. These materials are designed to release ions that promote the remineralization of tooth structure and stimulate the formation of secondary dentin. This property is particularly advantageous in treating early carious lesions, as bioactive materials can help to halt or reverse the carious process without the need for extensive removal of tooth structure. Additionally, bioactive materials contribute to a more natural healing process by enhancing the bond between the restoration and the tooth, which can improve the longevity of the restoration and reduce the likelihood of secondary caries.

Recent developments have also focused on enhancing the adhesion properties of dental materials. Advances in adhesive technology have led to the creation of more effective bonding agents that provide stronger and more reliable adhesion between composite resins or ceramics and the tooth structure. Modern adhesive systems often incorporate new types of monomers and improved formulations that enhance the bond strength while minimizing the potential for post-operative sensitivity. These improvements ensure that restorations remain securely bonded to the tooth structure, thereby increasing the durability and success rates of minimally invasive treatments.

In addition to these specific material innovations, the integration of digital technologies has revolutionized the use of biomaterials in minimally invasive dentistry. Digital impression systems, for instance, allow for the precise and non-invasive capture of tooth and oral cavity morphology. This digital data can then be used to design restorations with high accuracy, ensuring a better fit and reducing the need for adjustments. CAD/CAM (computer-aided design and computer-aided manufacturing) technology further complements these advances by enabling the creation of custom restorations with a high degree of precision and efficiency. The combination of digital impressions and CAD/CAM technology enhances the overall workflow, from diagnosis and treatment planning to the final restoration, contributing to better clinical outcomes and patient satisfaction.

The ongoing research and development in biomaterials also address the need for materials that are biocompatible and have minimal impact on the environment. Modern biomaterials are increasingly designed to be more biocompatible, reducing the risk of allergic reactions and ensuring that they interact harmoniously with the oral tissues. Additionally, there is a growing emphasis on the sustainability of dental materials, with efforts focused on developing materials that are both effective and environmentally friendly. This includes the exploration of recyclable or biodegradable materials and the reduction of harmful byproducts during the manufacturing process.

In conclusion, innovations in biomaterials are integral to the advancement of minimally invasive dentistry. The continuous evolution of composite resins, dental ceramics, bioactive materials, and adhesive technologies reflects a commitment to improving the quality and effectiveness of dental restorations while preserving as much natural tooth structure as possible. The integration of digital tools further enhances the precision and efficiency of these materials, leading to better clinical outcomes and greater patient satisfaction. As research and technology continue to advance, the field of minimally invasive dentistry will benefit from even more refined and effective biomaterials, ensuring that dental care remains both cutting-edge and patient-centered.

The integration of advanced biomaterials into minimally invasive dentistry has led to significant improvements in both clinical outcomes and patient satisfaction. As we explore these innovations, it becomes evident that the continual evolution of materials plays a crucial role in enhancing the effectiveness and appeal of minimally invasive procedures.

A prominent area of innovation lies in the development of advanced composite resins. The introduction of nano- and micro-hybrid composites has markedly enhanced the performance of these materials. Nano-filled composites, for example, incorporate nanoparticles that improve the material's mechanical properties, such as its hardness and wear resistance. These composites offer superior polishability, which contributes to their resistance to staining and discoloration, a critical factor in maintaining the aesthetic quality of restorations over time. Additionally, the reduced particle size allows for a smoother surface and better adaptation to tooth structures, which is essential in achieving a seamless integration of the restoration with the natural tooth.

In parallel, the refinement of dental ceramics has significantly impacted the field of minimally invasive dentistry. The evolution from traditional, opaque ceramics to high-translucency materials like lithium disilicate has allowed for the creation of restorations that closely mimic the natural appearance of teeth. Lithium disilicate ceramics, known for their exceptional strength and aesthetic qualities, have become a preferred choice for applications such as veneers, crowns, and inlays. These materials can be manufactured in ultra-thin layers, reducing the need for extensive tooth preparation and preserving more of the original tooth structure. This advancement not only enhances the aesthetic outcome but also aligns with the principles of minimally invasive dentistry by prioritizing tooth preservation.

The development of zirconia ceramics represents another significant leap forward. Zirconia, with its high fracture toughness and strength, is particularly beneficial for posterior restorations where durability is paramount. Recent advances have also introduced translucent zirconia variants, bridging the gap between strength and aesthetics. These innovations allow for the use of zirconia in a broader range of clinical scenarios, including both anterior and posterior restorations, while maintaining a natural look that complements the surrounding dentition.

Bioactive materials have emerged as a groundbreaking development in minimally invasive dentistry, offering a dynamic approach to dental restoration and repair. Bioactive glasses and calcium silicate-based materials, such as mineral trioxide aggregate (MTA), have been designed to actively interact with dental tissues. These materials release beneficial ions that encourage remineralization of the tooth structure and support the formation of secondary dentin. This bioactivity is particularly advantageous in treating early carious lesions and in situations where the preservation of tooth vitality is essential. By promoting natural healing processes and enhancing the bond between the restoration and the tooth, bioactive materials contribute to the long-term success of minimally invasive treatments.

Additionally, advances in adhesive technology have played a crucial role in the success of minimally invasive restorations. Modern adhesive systems have been developed to provide stronger, more reliable bonds between restorative materials and tooth structures. The introduction of universal adhesives, which can bond to various substrates including enamel, dentin, and ceramics, simplifies the clinical workflow and improves the predictability of adhesion. These adhesives are formulated with improved monomers that enhance bond strength and reduce the potential for post-operative sensitivity, leading to more stable and durable restorations.

The role of digital technology in supporting these material innovations cannot be overstated. Digital impression systems, for example, offer a non-invasive and highly accurate method for capturing the details of the tooth and surrounding structures. This digital data is then used to design and fabricate restorations with precision, resulting in a better fit and reduced need for adjustments. The integration of CAD/CAM technology further enhances this process by allowing for the creation of custom restorations with high accuracy and efficiency. These technologies not only streamline the workflow but also contribute to the overall success and longevity of minimally invasive treatments.

Moreover, the emphasis on biocompatibility and sustainability in material development reflects a growing awareness of the need for materials that are safe for patients and environmentally responsible. Innovations in this area include the development of materials that minimize allergic reactions and the exploration of recyclable or biodegradable options. This focus on biocompatibility and environmental impact aligns with the broader goals of modern dentistry, which seeks to provide effective care while minimizing potential harm to patients and the planet.

In summary, the advancements in biomaterials for minimally invasive dentistry represent a significant evolution in dental practice. The continuous improvement of composite resins, ceramics, and bioactive materials, coupled with enhanced adhesive technologies and digital tools, has transformed the landscape of restorative dentistry. These innovations not only enhance the durability and aesthetics of restorations but also adhere to the principles of minimally invasive dentistry by prioritizing tooth preservation and promoting patient-centered care. As the field continues to advance, the integration of these cutting-edge materials and technologies will undoubtedly lead to even more refined and effective minimally invasive treatment options.

The integration of recent innovations in biomaterials into minimally invasive dentistry has brought about transformative changes in clinical practice, enhancing the effectiveness and appeal of restorative procedures. These advancements not only address the functional needs of dental restorations but also cater to the growing demand for aesthetics and patient comfort. The focus on biomaterials that support minimally invasive techniques underscores a commitment to preserving natural tooth structure while delivering durable and aesthetically pleasing outcomes.

Recent developments in composite resins have significantly improved their performance in minimally invasive treatments. One of the key innovations is the introduction of resin composites with improved mechanical properties and wear resistance. Modern composites often incorporate advanced filler technologies, such as microhybrid and nanohybrid systems, which enhance their strength and longevity. These fillers are engineered to offer superior resistance to wear and staining, thus maintaining the aesthetic quality of restorations over time. Furthermore, advances in polymer chemistry have led to the creation of composites with better bonding capabilities to both enamel and dentin. This ensures a more secure adhesion, which is crucial in minimizing the risk of restoration failure and reducing postoperative sensitivity.

In addition to improvements in composite resins, significant strides have been made in the development of dental ceramics. These advancements include the enhancement of material properties such as translucency, strength, and biocompatibility. Lithium disilicate ceramics have gained prominence due to their exceptional strength and natural-looking translucency, making them suitable for a range of restorations from veneers to crowns. The material's ability to be fabricated into thin layers without compromising strength aligns with the principles of minimally invasive dentistry, as it allows for conservative tooth preparation while achieving excellent aesthetic results. Similarly, advancements in zirconia ceramics have introduced more translucent variants that bridge the gap between strength and aesthetics, expanding their use in anterior restorations.

Another notable innovation is the development of bioactive materials, which have introduced a new dimension to restorative dentistry. Bioactive materials, such as calcium silicate-based cements and bioactive glass, interact positively with tooth structure by releasing ions that promote remineralization and enhance the formation of secondary dentin. These materials are particularly beneficial in managing early carious lesions and in procedures where tooth preservation is paramount. The use of bioactive materials aligns with the minimally invasive approach by supporting the natural healing processes of the tooth and reducing the need for more invasive interventions.

The role of adhesive technologies has also advanced, further supporting the efficacy of minimally invasive techniques. Modern adhesive systems are designed to enhance the bond strength between restorative materials and tooth structures. Innovations include universal adhesives that simplify the bonding process by working effectively with various substrates, including enamel, dentin, and ceramics. These adhesives are formulated to reduce the incidence of postoperative sensitivity and improve the durability of restorations. The enhanced bonding capabilities of these adhesives contribute to the overall success of minimally invasive procedures by ensuring a strong and stable restoration.

The integration of digital technologies has revolutionized the use of biomaterials in minimally invasive dentistry. Digital impression systems, for instance, provide precise and non-invasive means of capturing tooth and tissue details, which are then used to design and fabricate restorations with high accuracy. The use of CAD/CAM technology allows for the efficient creation of custom restorations, which can be produced with a high degree of precision and minimal adjustment. This technology not only streamlines the clinical workflow but also enhances the fit and longevity of restorations, aligning with the goals of minimally invasive dentistry.

Additionally, the emphasis on biocompatibility and environmental sustainability in the development of biomaterials reflects a growing awareness of the broader impact of dental practices. Efforts to create materials that are less likely to cause allergic reactions and that incorporate sustainable practices underscore a commitment to patient safety and environmental responsibility. Innovations in this area include the development of materials that minimize waste and are recyclable or biodegradable, contributing to a more sustainable approach to dental care.

In conclusion, the innovations in biomaterials for minimally invasive dentistry represent a significant advancement in the field, improving both the functionality and aesthetics of dental restorations. The development of advanced composite resins, enhanced dental ceramics, and bioactive materials, along with improved adhesive technologies and digital tools, has transformed restorative dentistry by making procedures less invasive while achieving better clinical outcomes. As the field continues to evolve, these innovations will undoubtedly lead to even more refined and effective minimally invasive treatments, enhancing patient care and satisfaction while upholding the principles of tooth preservation and aesthetic excellence.

CHAPTER 41: ADDRESSING COMMON MISCONCEPTIONS ABOUT MINIMALLY INVASIVE DENTISTRY

Minimally invasive dentistry represents a paradigm shift in the field, emphasizing procedures that preserve as much of the natural tooth structure as possible while delivering effective treatment outcomes. Despite its advancements and growing adoption, various misconceptions persist that can hinder its implementation and acceptance among patients and practitioners alike. This chapter aims to address and debunk these common misconceptions, providing clarity on the treatment effectiveness, patient outcomes, and practical applications of minimally invasive techniques.

One prevalent misconception about minimally invasive dentistry is that it is less effective than traditional, more invasive methods. This belief often stems from a lack of familiarity with the advancements in materials and techniques that have significantly enhanced the effectiveness of minimally invasive approaches. Minimally invasive techniques are designed to be highly effective by targeting the root causes of dental issues while preserving as much of the natural tooth as possible. For instance, in the case of carious lesions, minimal intervention strategies such as selective carious tissue removal and the use of bioactive materials can halt the progression of decay and promote natural remineralization. These methods are supported by extensive clinical research that demonstrates their efficacy in managing dental caries and other conditions, thereby challenging the notion that less invasive approaches are inherently inferior.

Another common misunderstanding is that minimally invasive procedures are only suitable for simple or superficial dental issues. This misconception overlooks the versatility of minimally invasive techniques, which are applicable to a broad spectrum of dental conditions. For example, advancements in adhesive dentistry and the development of high-strength materials have made it possible to perform minimally invasive restorations for more complex cases, including extensive dental damage and aesthetic improvements. Modern techniques such as resin infiltration for early carious lesions or the use of CAD/CAM technology for precise restorations allow for effective management of both simple and complex dental issues with minimal impact on healthy tooth structure.

A related myth is that minimally invasive procedures are less durable than traditional treatments. This belief can be attributed to the historical association of less invasive techniques with weaker materials and less robust outcomes. However, recent advancements in biomaterials have significantly improved the durability and longevity of minimally invasive restorations. Innovations in composite resins, dental ceramics, and bioactive materials have led to the development of highly durable and aesthetically pleasing restorations that can withstand the demands of daily function. These materials are designed to closely mimic the properties of natural teeth, providing long-lasting solutions that challenge the outdated perception that minimal invasiveness equates to reduced durability.

Patients may also harbor concerns that minimally invasive techniques are more costly compared to traditional methods. This perception often arises from the initial cost of advanced materials and technologies used in minimally invasive procedures. While it is true that some minimally invasive treatments may have higher upfront costs, these expenses should be weighed against the long-term benefits. Minimally invasive techniques often result in fewer complications, reduced need for follow-up treatments, and less extensive future interventions. These factors contribute to overall cost-effectiveness by minimizing the need for more extensive and costly treatments in the future, thus offering a value proposition that aligns with long-term patient care and oral health management.

Another misconception is that minimally invasive dentistry is only relevant for cosmetic or elective procedures. This view fails to recognize the essential role that minimally invasive techniques play in preventive and restorative care. For instance, early intervention strategies using minimal intervention can prevent the progression of dental diseases and reduce the need for more invasive treatments. Techniques such as fluoride application, sealants, and remineralization therapies are integral components of a minimally invasive approach that focuses on preserving tooth health and preventing significant dental issues. By emphasizing prevention and early intervention, minimally invasive dentistry addresses fundamental aspects of oral health that extend beyond purely cosmetic concerns.

Additionally, there is a belief that minimally invasive dentistry requires highly specialized training and is therefore impractical for general practitioners. While it is true that some minimally invasive techniques may require additional training and expertise, many of these methods are designed to be integrated into routine dental practice. Continuous advancements in dental education and technology have made it increasingly feasible for general practitioners to adopt minimally invasive techniques. With proper training and access to modern tools and materials, practitioners can effectively incorporate these techniques into their practice, expanding their capabilities and offering a wider range of treatments to their patients.

In conclusion, addressing and debunking these common misconceptions is crucial for advancing the practice of minimally invasive dentistry. By clarifying the effectiveness of these techniques, their applicability to various dental conditions, and their long-term benefits, it becomes evident that minimally invasive dentistry offers a valuable approach to patient care. As dental professionals and patients gain a clearer understanding of the capabilities and advantages of minimally invasive techniques, the potential for improved oral health outcomes and patient satisfaction will continue to grow, reinforcing the importance of embracing and advancing this progressive approach in modern dental practice.

The discussion on addressing misconceptions about minimally invasive dentistry requires a deeper examination of its practical applications and outcomes to effectively dispel prevalent misunderstandings. One area where misconceptions often arise is in the perception of the complexity and time requirements associated with minimally invasive procedures. There is a belief that such techniques are time-consuming and complex compared to traditional methods. This perception stems from a lack of familiarity with the streamlined protocols and advanced technologies that minimize procedural time and complexity.

In reality, many minimally invasive techniques are designed

to be efficient and less time-consuming. For example, the use of modern adhesive systems and simplified cavity preparation techniques has significantly reduced the time required for procedures such as composite restorations. Advances in technology, including the integration of digital tools and CAD/CAM systems, have further streamlined the process, allowing for more precise and faster restorations. These technologies enable practitioners to achieve high-quality results in a shorter time frame, challenging the notion that minimally invasive methods are inherently more complex or time-consuming.

Another misconception relates to the perceived necessity of extensive prior diagnostic work and preparatory steps before minimally invasive treatment can be administered. Some believe that such preparatory work makes minimally invasive procedures less practical or less straightforward compared to more traditional approaches. However, this misconception overlooks the fact that thorough diagnostics and preparation are crucial for all effective dental treatments, whether invasive or minimally invasive. The use of advanced diagnostic tools such as digital radiography and intraoral cameras enhances the accuracy of assessments, thereby improving treatment planning and outcomes. These technologies facilitate a more precise and informed approach to patient care, demonstrating that the preparatory steps in minimally invasive dentistry are integral to achieving optimal results.

A related concern is that minimally invasive techniques require a significant investment in new technologies and materials, which can be perceived as a barrier to adoption. While it is true that initial costs for advanced technologies and high-quality biomaterials can be substantial, it is important to consider the long-term benefits and cost-effectiveness of these investments. Minimally invasive techniques often lead to fewer complications and reduced need for extensive follow-up treatments, ultimately resulting in cost savings over time. The long-term benefits of improved patient outcomes, reduced procedural costs, and enhanced efficiency should be weighed against the initial investment, highlighting the value of incorporating these techniques into practice.

Patients sometimes harbor the misconception that minimally invasive treatments are not as durable or long-lasting as traditional methods. This belief is often rooted in outdated views of early minimally invasive technologies, which may have had limitations in durability and longevity. However, advancements in biomaterials and bonding technologies have significantly improved the durability and lifespan of minimally invasive restorations. Modern composites, ceramics, and other materials are engineered to withstand the forces of daily use while maintaining aesthetic appeal. Clinical studies and long-term outcomes consistently demonstrate that well-executed minimally invasive treatments can offer comparable, if not superior, durability to traditional methods.

Another significant misconception is that minimally invasive dentistry is only applicable to certain types of patients or specific conditions. Some may believe that these techniques are not suitable for complex or severe dental issues. This view underestimates the versatility and adaptability of minimally invasive approaches. While these techniques are indeed effective for early intervention and preventive care, they are also applicable to a range of restorative scenarios. For instance, advanced minimally invasive techniques such as laser dentistry and micro-invasive restorations have proven effective in treating more complex dental conditions, including substantial carious lesions and extensive tooth damage. The adaptability of minimally invasive approaches allows for tailored treatment plans that address a wide array of patient needs.

Furthermore, misconceptions about the training and

expertise required for minimally invasive dentistry can deter practitioners from exploring these methods. Some may assume that these techniques necessitate extensive specialized training beyond the reach of general practitioners. In reality, many minimally invasive procedures are designed to be integrated into routine dental practice with proper training and continuing education. Advances in dental education and resources have made it increasingly feasible for general practitioners to acquire the skills and knowledge needed to implement minimally invasive techniques effectively. Access to professional development opportunities and educational resources helps bridge the gap between traditional and minimally invasive practices, fostering broader adoption and implementation.

Addressing these misconceptions involves not only clarifying the capabilities and benefits of minimally invasive techniques but also emphasizing the importance of ongoing education and evidence-based practice. By understanding the realities of minimally invasive dentistry and its practical applications, both practitioners and patients can make informed decisions that enhance oral health outcomes and promote the adoption of innovative and effective treatment approaches. The evolution of dental practice towards minimally invasive methods represents a significant advancement in patient care, guided by the principles of preservation, precision, and long-term health benefits.

One prevalent misconception about minimally invasive dentistry is that it is only suitable for certain demographic groups or specific types of dental conditions. This view can be misleading, as minimally invasive techniques are not restricted by age, the severity of dental issues, or the complexity of cases. For instance, while it is true that early-stage carious lesions are ideal candidates for minimally invasive treatments such as fluoride varnishes or resin infiltrations, these techniques can also be effectively employed in more complex situations. Advanced minimally invasive approaches, including laser therapy and micro-mineralization techniques, have demonstrated efficacy in managing severe carious lesions and extensive tooth damage. The flexibility and adaptability of minimally invasive methods make them applicable across a broad spectrum of patient needs, debunking the notion that these approaches are limited in scope.

Another misconception involves the belief that minimally invasive dentistry is synonymous with lesser clinical outcomes. There is a concern among some patients and practitioners that the less invasive nature of these techniques might compromise the quality or longevity of the results. However, evidence from numerous clinical studies and long-term research consistently shows that minimally invasive treatments can achieve outcomes that are comparable to, or even exceed, those of more traditional methods. Innovations in biomaterials and techniques have significantly enhanced the durability and effectiveness of minimally invasive procedures. For instance, the development of advanced composite resins and high-strength dental ceramics has bolstered the longevity and performance of restorations, proving that these methods do not sacrifice quality for conservativeness.

The misconception that minimally invasive techniques are less cost-effective than traditional methods also warrants attention. Some practitioners and patients may assume that the initial investment in advanced technologies and materials used in minimally invasive dentistry translates into higher costs, making these approaches seem economically unfeasible. In reality, the cost-effectiveness of minimally invasive dentistry often becomes evident over the long term. The reduced need for extensive follow-up treatments, fewer complications, and lower rates of restorative failure contribute to overall cost savings. The emphasis on prevention and early intervention not only minimizes the need for more invasive procedures but also fosters better long-term oral health outcomes, thereby reducing the overall financial burden on both patients and dental practices.

Another significant misunderstanding is related to the level of skill and training required to perform minimally invasive procedures. There is a belief that these techniques necessitate highly specialized training and are therefore inaccessible to general practitioners. While it is true that some minimally invasive techniques require specific training, many procedures are designed to be integrated into general dental practice with appropriate education and practice. Continuing education programs and professional development opportunities are widely available, enabling general practitioners to acquire the necessary skills to implement minimally invasive techniques effectively. The growing availability of these educational resources underscores the feasibility of incorporating these approaches into routine dental care.

Additionally, patients often have misconceptions about the immediacy and invasiveness of treatment outcomes. Some believe that minimally invasive procedures offer temporary solutions rather than long-lasting results. This belief is not supported by current evidence, which shows that when properly executed, minimally invasive techniques provide durable and effective solutions for various dental conditions. For example, minimally invasive restorations such as tooth-colored composites and ultra-thin veneers offer both aesthetic and functional benefits, with results that can endure for many years when properly maintained. The durability of these treatments is further supported by advancements in materials science and adhesive technologies, which enhance the longevity of minimally invasive restorations.

Misunderstandings about the role of patient compliance in

the success of minimally invasive treatments also need addressing. Some might assume that these techniques are effective regardless of patient adherence to recommended care protocols. In truth, the success of minimally invasive treatments heavily relies on patient engagement and adherence to oral hygiene practices. Educating patients about the importance of maintaining good oral hygiene, attending regular check-ups, and following post-treatment instructions is crucial for maximizing the benefits of minimally invasive care. Effective communication and patient education are essential components in ensuring that patients understand their role in the long-term success of their treatments.

Finally, it is important to challenge the misconception that minimally invasive dentistry is merely a passing trend rather than a well-established and evidence-based approach. The growing body of research and clinical evidence supporting the effectiveness and benefits of minimally invasive techniques highlights their legitimacy and value in modern dental practice. The principles of minimally invasive dentistry—such as preserving tooth structure, enhancing patient comfort, and employing preventive measures—are grounded in sound scientific research and have been embraced by dental professionals worldwide.

In summary, addressing and debunking misconceptions about minimally invasive dentistry involves clarifying the practical applications, effectiveness, and economic value of these techniques. By understanding the true nature of minimally invasive practices, both patients and practitioners can better appreciate their role in enhancing dental care and improving oral health outcomes. As the field of dentistry continues to evolve, the integration of minimally invasive approaches represents a forward-thinking shift towards more conservative, patient-centered care.

CHAPTER 42: MINIMALLY INVASIVE TECHNIQUES IN COSMETIC DENTISTRY

In the realm of cosmetic dentistry, the shift towards minimally invasive techniques marks a significant evolution in enhancing patients' smiles while preserving the natural integrity of their teeth. This chapter delves into the application of these techniques, exploring procedures such as tooth whitening, aesthetic bonding, and veneers. The emphasis is on how these methods achieve aesthetically pleasing results while minimizing the need for extensive and potentially damaging dental interventions.

Tooth whitening, a staple in cosmetic dentistry, exemplifies the benefits of minimally invasive techniques. Traditionally, whitening procedures involved the use of strong chemicals and potentially aggressive methods to achieve desired results. However, modern advancements have shifted towards approaches that prioritize patient safety and comfort while still delivering effective outcomes. Contemporary tooth whitening systems use advanced formulations and delivery mechanisms to enhance the whitening effect while minimizing tooth sensitivity and enamel damage. For instance, the use of carbamide peroxide and hydrogen peroxide in lower concentrations, combined with custom-fitted trays or LED light activation, allows for a more controlled and gradual whitening process. This approach reduces the risk of adverse effects and provides a more comfortable experience for patients.

Aesthetic bonding is another technique that aligns with the principles of minimally invasive cosmetic dentistry. This procedure involves the application of tooth-colored resin materials to address various aesthetic concerns, such as minor chips, cracks, or gaps between teeth. Unlike traditional restorative methods that often require significant alteration of the tooth structure, aesthetic bonding is designed to be conservative. The process typically involves the etching of the tooth surface to enhance adhesion, followed by the application of the resin material, which is then sculpted and polished to achieve a natural appearance. The benefits of aesthetic bonding include its ability to provide immediate results with minimal alteration to the tooth structure, making it an ideal choice for patients seeking subtle enhancements without extensive dental work.

Veneers, particularly those made from advanced ceramic materials, represent a sophisticated application of minimally invasive techniques in cosmetic dentistry. Veneers are ultra-thin shells that are bonded to the front surface of the teeth to correct imperfections such as discoloration, unevenness, or slight misalignments. Traditional veneer procedures often required substantial removal of tooth enamel to accommodate the veneer, which could compromise the tooth's long-term health. Modern advancements have led to the development of veneers that are both thinner and stronger, allowing for a more conservative approach. Minimal preparation veneers, also known as no-prep veneers, require little to no removal of tooth structure, thereby preserving the natural tooth while still achieving dramatic cosmetic improvements. These veneers are custom-crafted to fit precisely and provide a natural appearance, making them a popular choice among patients seeking a less invasive solution for enhancing their smile.

The integration of digital technologies into cosmetic dentistry further underscores the benefits of minimally invasive techniques. Digital impressions and 3D imaging allow for precise planning and customization of cosmetic treatments. For example, digital smile design tools enable practitioners to visualize and plan the outcomes of aesthetic procedures before they begin, ensuring that the final result aligns with the patient's expectations. This technology not only enhances the accuracy of cosmetic interventions but also minimizes the need for trial and error, reducing the time and number of adjustments required to achieve the desired results.

Furthermore, advances in material science have contributed to the success of minimally invasive cosmetic procedures. Modern dental materials, including high-strength composites and ceramics, offer superior aesthetic qualities and durability. These materials are designed to blend seamlessly with natural teeth while resisting stains and wear, thus providing long-lasting results. The use of these advanced materials allows for conservative treatment options that do not compromise the tooth's structural integrity, ensuring that patients benefit from both aesthetic improvements and long-term dental health.

The principles of minimally invasive cosmetic dentistry are also reflected in the focus on patient-centered care. By prioritizing procedures that require less alteration of the natural tooth structure, cosmetic dentists can offer solutions that are both effective and conservative. This approach aligns with the growing emphasis on preventive and patient-centered dental care, where the goal is to achieve optimal results while preserving the natural health and function of the teeth.

In summary, the application of minimally invasive techniques in cosmetic dentistry represents a significant advancement in achieving aesthetic goals while minimizing the impact on tooth structure. Procedures such as tooth whitening, aesthetic bonding, and veneers illustrate how modern techniques can provide dramatic cosmetic enhancements with a conservative approach. The integration of digital technologies and advanced materials further supports the efficacy and appeal of these minimally invasive methods, ensuring that patients receive high-quality care with optimal outcomes. As cosmetic dentistry continues to evolve, the principles of minimally invasive techniques will remain central to delivering both beautiful and health-conscious dental solutions.

In examining the application of minimally invasive techniques within cosmetic dentistry, it is essential to delve deeper into how these methods align with contemporary standards of aesthetic treatment while maintaining a conservative approach to tooth preservation. These techniques, including tooth whitening, aesthetic bonding, and veneers, exemplify a shift towards approaches that not only enhance cosmetic outcomes but also prioritize the preservation of the natural dental structure.

Tooth whitening remains one of the most sought-after cosmetic procedures, largely due to its effectiveness and non-invasiveness. Modern whitening techniques leverage advanced formulations that enhance the safety and efficacy of the treatment. The use of peroxide-based gels, which are activated by light or heat, has been refined to reduce the risk of tooth sensitivity and gum irritation, common issues associated with earlier whitening methods. Additionally, at-home whitening kits, which often feature lower concentrations of active ingredients, provide a gradual and controlled approach to whitening. These kits, when used under professional guidance, can achieve significant results with minimal risk. The evolution of these products reflects a broader trend towards patient-centered care, where the goal is to maximize cosmetic benefit while minimizing potential discomfort.

Aesthetic bonding offers another avenue for achieving cosmetic improvements with minimal invasiveness. This procedure involves the application of a tooth-colored composite resin to correct minor imperfections such as small fractures, chips, or gaps. The process begins with the preparation of the tooth surface, which involves light etching to create a rough surface that enhances the bond between the resin and the tooth. The resin is then carefully applied, shaped, and cured using a special light to harden it. The bonding material is subsequently polished to match the natural tooth surface. This technique is particularly advantageous for patients seeking immediate results with minimal alteration to their existing tooth structure. The durability and adaptability of modern bonding materials also contribute to their success in achieving long-lasting and aesthetically pleasing outcomes.

Veneers represent a sophisticated application of minimally invasive techniques in cosmetic dentistry. These ultra-thin shells, typically crafted from porcelain or advanced composite materials, are bonded to the front surfaces of teeth to address a variety of aesthetic concerns, including discoloration, misalignment, and irregularities in tooth shape. Traditionally, the placement of veneers required substantial reduction of tooth enamel, which could compromise the tooth's health. However, advancements in veneer technology have introduced options such as minimal-prep or no-prep veneers, which require less invasive preparation. These modern veneers are designed to be ultra-thin yet highly durable, allowing for significant cosmetic enhancement with minimal removal of tooth structure. The precision in crafting these veneers is achieved through the use of digital impressions and computer-aided design (CAD), ensuring a perfect fit and natural appearance.

The integration of digital tools into cosmetic procedures has revolutionized the field of minimally invasive dentistry. Digital imaging and 3D scanning provide accurate representations of the dental structure, enabling precise planning and execution of cosmetic treatments. For instance, digital smile design technology allows clinicians to create virtual simulations of the expected results before any physical alterations are made. This approach not only enhances patient satisfaction by providing a clear visualization of the outcome but also minimizes the need for multiple adjustments during the treatment process. The use of these technologies aligns with the principles of minimally invasive dentistry by ensuring that interventions are as accurate and conservative as possible.

Advancements in biomaterials also play a crucial role in the effectiveness of minimally invasive cosmetic procedures. Modern composite resins and dental ceramics are designed to offer superior aesthetic properties, including color matching and translucency, which closely mimic natural tooth enamel. These materials are also engineered to withstand the forces of daily chewing while resisting staining and wear. The development of such high-performance materials enables cosmetic dentists to perform treatments that not only achieve the desired visual results but also ensure durability and longevity.

The principles of minimally invasive cosmetic dentistry also emphasize patient comfort and safety. By opting for procedures that require less invasive preparation and utilize advanced materials and technologies, dentists can offer treatments that enhance the appearance of the teeth without compromising their structural integrity. This approach aligns with the broader goals of cosmetic dentistry, which aim to provide effective, long-lasting results while maintaining the overall health and functionality of the teeth.

In conclusion, minimally invasive techniques in cosmetic dentistry represent a significant advancement in the pursuit of aesthetic excellence. Procedures such as tooth whitening, aesthetic bonding, and veneers illustrate the shift towards methods that achieve desirable cosmetic outcomes with minimal disruption to the natural tooth structure. The integration of digital technologies and advanced biomaterials further supports the efficacy and appeal of these techniques, ensuring that patients receive high-quality care that prioritizes both aesthetic enhancement and dental health. As the field continues to evolve, the principles of minimally invasive dentistry will remain central to delivering cosmetic solutions that are both effective and conservative.

In the realm of cosmetic dentistry, minimally invasive techniques not only enhance aesthetic outcomes but also align with the principles of preserving natural tooth structure and ensuring patient comfort. The ongoing evolution in these techniques has paved the way for more conservative approaches that achieve significant cosmetic improvements while reducing the need for extensive alterations to the teeth.

One of the key areas where minimally invasive methods have made substantial strides is in the realm of tooth whitening. Historically, tooth whitening procedures often involved strong bleaching agents and techniques that could sometimes cause discomfort or damage to the enamel. Modern advancements, however, have refined these methods to improve safety and efficacy. Current whitening treatments utilize peroxide-based gels with controlled concentrations, activated by either light or laser technology. This controlled activation minimizes the potential for enamel damage and reduces sensitivity, a common side effect of older whitening systems. Additionally, the development of remineralizing agents that are included in some whitening products helps to counteract potential demineralization of the tooth structure, thus maintaining enamel integrity while achieving brighter teeth.

Aesthetic bonding, another pillar of minimally invasive cosmetic dentistry, has also undergone significant advancements. The evolution of composite resins has led to materials that not only offer excellent color match and translucency but also possess improved mechanical properties. These resins are now more resistant to staining and wear, enhancing their durability and making them more suitable for a variety of cosmetic applications. The bonding procedure itself has been optimized to be less invasive, involving minimal alteration to the tooth structure. This technique is particularly effective for addressing minor imperfections, such as small chips or gaps, without the need for more invasive procedures like crowns or veneers.

The application of veneers has similarly been revolutionized by minimally invasive approaches. Traditionally, veneer placement required significant reduction of the tooth's natural structure to accommodate the veneer. However, advances in veneer technology, including the development of ultra-thin and no-prep veneers, have significantly altered this approach. These modern veneers require minimal to no removal of tooth enamel, preserving the underlying tooth structure while still achieving a dramatic improvement in aesthetics. The precision involved in crafting these veneers is enhanced by digital technology, which allows for highly accurate impressions and designs. This ensures that the veneers fit perfectly and match the natural tooth color, providing a seamless and aesthetically pleasing result.

In addition to these advancements, the integration of digital tools and technologies has further enhanced the minimally invasive approach to cosmetic dentistry. Digital imaging and computer-aided design (CAD) play a crucial role in planning and executing cosmetic procedures. These technologies provide detailed and precise images of the dental structures, enabling clinicians to create highly accurate and customized treatment plans. For instance, digital smile design software allows for virtual simulations of potential outcomes, giving patients a clear view of the expected results before any actual treatment begins. This level of precision not only improves the accuracy of the procedures but also enhances patient satisfaction by ensuring that the final results align closely with the patient's expectations.

Furthermore, the use of laser technology in cosmetic procedures has contributed to the minimally invasive philosophy by offering highly precise and controlled interventions. Lasers can be used for various purposes, including gum contouring, stain removal, and even the application of certain bonding materials. The precision of laser treatment minimizes the impact on surrounding tissues, reduces the need for traditional surgical methods, and often leads to faster healing times and less discomfort for the patient.

The shift towards minimally invasive techniques in cosmetic dentistry also reflects a broader trend towards patient-centered care. Patients today are increasingly informed and concerned about the long-term effects of dental treatments, including the preservation of their natural teeth. Minimally invasive approaches address these concerns by focusing on achieving cosmetic improvements while maintaining the health and integrity of the teeth. This approach not only meets the aesthetic goals of patients but also aligns with the principles of conservative dental practice.

As minimally invasive techniques continue to evolve, the

integration of new materials, technologies, and treatment methodologies will further enhance the capabilities of cosmetic dentistry. The emphasis on preserving natural tooth structure, improving patient comfort, and achieving superior aesthetic outcomes remains central to the field. By leveraging these advancements, cosmetic dentists can offer treatments that not only enhance the appearance of the teeth but also uphold the fundamental principles of minimally invasive care. This ongoing innovation ensures that patients receive the highest standard of care while benefiting from the latest advancements in dental technology and materials.

CHAPTER 43: EVALUATING OUTCOMES AND SUCCESS RATES IN MINIMALLY INVASIVE DENTISTRY

The evaluation of outcomes and success rates in minimally invasive dentistry is crucial for understanding the efficacy of these treatments and ensuring high standards of care. This chapter delves into the methodologies employed to track the effectiveness of minimally invasive procedures, assess patient satisfaction, and use clinical data to refine and improve practice.

To begin with, assessing the effectiveness of minimally invasive treatments involves a combination of objective and subjective measures. Clinically, the success of these treatments is often evaluated through follow-up examinations that monitor the stability and durability of the results. For instance, in the case of minimally invasive restorations such as dental sealants or composite fillings, long-term follow-up is essential to assess issues such as wear, discoloration, and the integrity of the bond. Invasive techniques that focus on preserving natural tooth structure demand thorough and repeated evaluations to ensure that the intended outcomes, such as prevention of caries progression or correction of aesthetic imperfections, are achieved.

Objective measures include the use of advanced diagnostic tools such as digital radiography, which allows for precise imaging of restorations and underlying tooth structures. These images can help detect any early signs of failure, such as leakage around restorations or changes in the underlying tooth structure. The accuracy of these tools helps in making timely interventions if any issues are identified. Additionally, the use of clinical indices, such as the modified Ryge criteria, helps in systematically evaluating restorations based on parameters such as marginal integrity, surface texture, and color match.

Subjective assessments, on the other hand, involve evaluating patient-reported outcomes, which are increasingly recognized as vital components of treatment success. Patient satisfaction surveys, interviews, and questionnaires provide insights into the perceived effectiveness of the treatment, comfort levels, and overall satisfaction with the results. These subjective measures can reveal aspects of the treatment experience that are not captured through clinical evaluations alone, such as the impact on daily life, functional outcomes, and aesthetic satisfaction. For example, a patient who has undergone tooth whitening might report not only on the improvement in tooth color but also on any associated sensitivity or changes in their self-confidence.

Tracking success rates also involves examining failure rates and identifying factors that contribute to suboptimal outcomes. Analyzing data from various cases helps in understanding patterns that may indicate common issues or risks associated with certain treatments. For example, a higher failure rate in a specific type of restoration might prompt a review of the materials used, the technique employed, or the patient's compliance with aftercare instructions. Identifying these patterns allows for the refinement of techniques and materials, improving overall success rates and patient outcomes.

The integration of digital tools plays a significant role in refining practices and improving success rates. Electronic health records (EHRs) and practice management software enable comprehensive data collection and analysis, facilitating the tracking of treatment outcomes over time. Data analytics can identify trends, compare outcomes across different patient demographics, and evaluate the effectiveness of various treatment protocols. For instance, tracking the longevity of minimally invasive fillings across different age groups or dental conditions can provide valuable insights into how well these treatments perform under varying circumstances.

Moreover, continuous professional development and evidence-based practice are crucial for improving outcomes. Staying abreast of the latest research, innovations in materials, and advancements in techniques ensures that practitioners are utilizing the most effective methods available. Participating in professional organizations, attending conferences, and engaging in peer-reviewed research contribute to a deeper understanding of treatment outcomes and foster the adoption of best practices.

Patient education and involvement are also integral to the evaluation of outcomes. Ensuring that patients are well-informed about their treatments and their role in maintaining oral health can influence the success rates of minimally invasive procedures. Educated patients are more likely to follow aftercare instructions, adhere to preventive measures, and report any issues promptly, all of which contribute to better long-term outcomes.

In summary, evaluating outcomes and success rates in minimally invasive dentistry requires a comprehensive approach that incorporates both objective clinical measures and subjective patient feedback. By utilizing advanced diagnostic tools, systematic tracking methods, and data analysis, practitioners can gain a clearer understanding of treatment efficacy and refine their techniques to enhance patient care. The integration of digital tools, ongoing professional development, and effective patient education further supports the continuous improvement of minimally invasive dental practices, ultimately leading to better patient outcomes and satisfaction.

In evaluating the outcomes and success rates of minimally invasive dental treatments, a nuanced approach is required to capture the full scope of treatment efficacy and patient satisfaction. A crucial aspect of this evaluation involves the meticulous tracking of treatment effectiveness through a variety of clinical and subjective measures.

One of the fundamental methods for tracking treatment effectiveness is the systematic monitoring of clinical outcomes over time. This often involves regular follow-up appointments where the condition of the treated areas is assessed. For instance, in minimally invasive procedures such as dental sealants or conservative fillings, it is important to regularly check for any signs of deterioration or failure. Clinical evaluations might include visual inspections and the use of diagnostic tools such as bitewing radiographs or intraoral cameras, which help in detecting issues that may not be immediately visible. For example, radiographs can reveal underlying problems like secondary caries or changes in tooth structure that could indicate a potential failure of the restoration.

To ensure accuracy, practitioners often employ standardized criteria for evaluating the success of treatments. These criteria, which are based on clinical research and consensus guidelines, help in providing a consistent framework for assessing outcomes. For instance, the modified Ryge criteria, widely used for evaluating dental restorations, focus on parameters such as marginal adaptation, surface texture, and color match. Utilizing these criteria allows for a systematic and reproducible assessment of the treatment results, making it easier to compare outcomes across different cases and practitioners.

In addition to clinical evaluations, the assessment of patient satisfaction plays a significant role in evaluating treatment success. Patient feedback provides insights into the perceived effectiveness of the treatment and its impact on daily life. Surveys and questionnaires are commonly used tools to gather patient-reported outcomes. These instruments can address various aspects of the patient experience, including comfort during the procedure, ease of post-treatment maintenance, and overall satisfaction with the aesthetic results. Patient satisfaction is not only indicative of treatment success but also influences the patient's adherence to recommended follow-up care and preventive measures.

Analyzing patient feedback also helps in identifying areas where treatments may fall short of expectations. For example, if a significant number of patients report sensitivity or discomfort following a minimally invasive procedure, this could signal a need for refinement in technique or material selection. Understanding these patient experiences enables practitioners to make informed adjustments to their practice, thereby enhancing the overall quality of care.

Furthermore, the use of digital tools and data analytics has revolutionized the evaluation process in modern dentistry. Electronic health records (EHRs) and practice management software facilitate comprehensive data collection, enabling practitioners to track treatment outcomes across a large patient population. By aggregating data from multiple cases, practitioners can identify trends and patterns that inform their understanding of treatment success and failure rates. For example, data analysis might reveal that certain materials or techniques yield better long-term results in specific patient demographics or clinical conditions. This evidence-based approach allows for continuous improvement and the adoption of best practices in minimally invasive dentistry.

The integration of digital imaging technologies also plays a critical role in outcome evaluation. Advanced imaging techniques, such as cone beam computed tomography (CBCT), provide detailed three-dimensional views of the treated areas, offering a more comprehensive assessment of treatment success. These images can help in detecting subtle changes in tooth structure or the integrity of restorations that may not be visible with traditional two-dimensional radiographs. By incorporating these advanced imaging modalities, practitioners can gain a more accurate understanding of the effectiveness of minimally invasive treatments.

Moreover, longitudinal studies and research contribute significantly to evaluating the success rates of minimally invasive techniques. Research studies that follow patients over extended periods provide valuable data on the long-term outcomes of these treatments. These studies often involve collaboration between academic institutions and clinical practices, allowing for a broader evaluation of treatment efficacy and durability. Participation in or access to such research can help practitioners stay informed about the latest advancements and emerging trends in minimally invasive dentistry.

In conclusion, evaluating outcomes and success rates in minimally invasive dentistry involves a multifaceted approach that combines clinical assessments, patient feedback, and data analysis. By employing standardized evaluation criteria, gathering patient-reported outcomes, and utilizing advanced digital tools, practitioners can obtain a comprehensive understanding of treatment effectiveness. Continuous monitoring and analysis of these outcomes, supported by research and evidence-based practices, ensure that minimally invasive techniques are refined and optimized to meet the highest standards of care. This ongoing evaluation process is essential for maintaining and improving the quality of minimally invasive dental treatments, ultimately leading to better patient outcomes and enhanced satisfaction.

The evaluation of outcomes and success rates in minimally invasive dentistry extends beyond immediate clinical observations to encompass a broader spectrum of factors influencing long-term success. An integral aspect of this evaluation is the continuous refinement of techniques and materials based on accumulated clinical data and patient experiences.

A critical element in this process involves the analysis of treatment longevity and durability. Minimally invasive procedures often aim to preserve tooth structure and function while addressing dental issues conservatively. Therefore, monitoring the lifespan of restorations and the stability of treated areas over time is essential for assessing their long-term success. This entails not only regular follow-ups but also the systematic documentation of treatment outcomes in clinical records. For instance, practitioners might track the occurrence of secondary caries, restoration failures, or the need for retreatment. This data provides insights into the effectiveness of different materials and techniques, guiding future clinical decisions and practice improvements.

In addition to tracking clinical outcomes, a comprehensive approach to outcome evaluation includes assessing the functional and aesthetic success of treatments. Functional success refers to the restoration's ability to restore or maintain proper oral function, such as chewing and speaking. Aesthetically, it involves evaluating whether the treatment meets the patient's expectations in terms of appearance. Both aspects are crucial for determining the overall success of minimally invasive procedures. For example, a tooth-colored composite filling should not only blend seamlessly with the surrounding tooth structure but also withstand the mechanical stresses of daily use without degradation. Evaluating these parameters involves both subjective assessments by patients and objective evaluations by practitioners.

Patient feedback is instrumental in providing a holistic view of treatment outcomes. Collecting and analyzing this feedback helps identify trends and areas for improvement. For instance, patients might report issues such as post-treatment sensitivity or discomfort, which can indicate potential shortcomings in the treatment approach or materials used. By systematically addressing these concerns and making necessary adjustments, practitioners can enhance patient satisfaction and treatment efficacy. Moreover, patient satisfaction surveys can reveal insights into how well the treatment aligns with patient expectations, which can be crucial for improving patient communication and care strategies.

Another important consideration in evaluating success rates is the integration of evidence-based practices. Utilizing the latest research and clinical guidelines helps ensure that the techniques and materials used are based on the most current and robust evidence. This approach not only improves treatment outcomes but also supports the adoption of innovative practices that enhance patient care. For instance, research may reveal new advancements in biomaterials that offer improved durability or aesthetics, prompting practitioners to incorporate these innovations into their practice.

To further enhance outcome evaluation, dental practices increasingly employ data analytics and digital tools. Electronic health records (EHRs) and practice management software enable the collection and analysis of comprehensive patient data. These systems facilitate the identification of patterns and trends in treatment outcomes, allowing for data-driven decision-making. For example, data analysis might uncover correlations between specific materials or techniques and improved long-term outcomes, guiding practitioners toward more effective approaches.

Additionally, the role of clinical audits and peer reviews cannot be overstated. Regularly reviewing clinical cases and outcomes within a practice or through peer review processes helps identify best practices and areas for improvement. These reviews often involve evaluating a range of cases, assessing adherence to treatment protocols, and discussing cases with peers to gain different perspectives. This collaborative approach fosters a culture of continuous learning and improvement, ultimately benefiting patient care.

Finally, the integration of patient-centered care principles is vital in evaluating treatment success. Minimally invasive dentistry emphasizes the importance of patient involvement in treatment planning and decision-making. Engaging patients in their care not only improves their satisfaction but also contributes to better adherence to treatment recommendations and follow-up care. By prioritizing patient education and involvement, practitioners can ensure that treatments are tailored to individual needs and preferences, leading to more successful outcomes.

In conclusion, the evaluation of outcomes and success rates in minimally invasive dentistry is a multifaceted process that involves tracking clinical effectiveness, assessing patient satisfaction, and integrating evidence-based practices. By employing a comprehensive approach that includes clinical monitoring, patient feedback, data analysis, and continuous learning, practitioners can enhance the effectiveness and quality of minimally invasive treatments. This ongoing evaluation not only ensures that treatments are meeting their intended goals but also supports the advancement of minimally invasive dentistry through continuous refinement and innovation.

CHAPTER 44: THE FUTURE OF MINIMALLY INVASIVE DENTISTRY

The future of minimally invasive dentistry promises to be as transformative as its past has been. As we look ahead, several key trends and advancements are poised to shape the next era of dental care. These developments are not only enhancing the precision and effectiveness of treatments but are also fundamentally changing the way dental practices approach patient care.

One of the most promising areas of innovation is the advancement in digital technologies. Digital tools, such as intraoral scanners and 3D imaging systems, have already begun to revolutionize minimally invasive procedures by providing highly detailed, real-time visualizations of the oral cavity. Looking forward, we can expect these technologies to become even more sophisticated, integrating with artificial intelligence (AI) and machine learning to further refine diagnostic capabilities and treatment planning. For instance, AI algorithms could analyze vast amounts of patient data to predict potential issues before they become clinically significant, allowing for even more proactive and preventive approaches.

Another significant trend is the continued development of biomaterials. Recent innovations in composite resins and dental ceramics have enhanced the durability, aesthetic quality, and biocompatibility of restorative materials. Future advancements are likely to bring even more refined materials that can better mimic natural tooth structure and function while offering improved resistance to wear and environmental factors. The integration of nanotechnology into biomaterials is also on the horizon, potentially leading to materials with enhanced strength and self-healing properties.

Personalized medicine is also expected to play a growing role in minimally invasive dentistry. Advances in genomics and personalized diagnostics could allow for treatments that are tailored to the individual's genetic makeup and specific dental health needs. For example, genetic testing might reveal predispositions to certain dental conditions, enabling practitioners to offer highly customized preventive care strategies and treatments that are more effective and less invasive.

The emphasis on preventive care will continue to drive the evolution of minimally invasive techniques. With an increasing focus on maintaining oral health and preventing disease rather than treating it reactively, new tools and methodologies will likely emerge to support this shift. This includes advancements in preventive technologies, such as caries detection devices and fluoride-releasing materials, which can help in early detection and management of dental issues before they necessitate more invasive interventions.

Tele-dentistry is another area poised for growth. The rise of telehealth and virtual consultations has already made its mark on various healthcare sectors, and dentistry is no exception. Future developments in tele-dentistry could enable more effective remote monitoring of dental health, real-time consultations, and even the implementation of certain preventive and diagnostic procedures from a distance. This could greatly enhance access to dental care, particularly for patients in underserved or remote areas.

Education and training for dental professionals will also evolve to keep pace with these advancements. As minimally invasive techniques become more complex and technology-driven, dental education will need to adapt accordingly. Future dental curricula may increasingly incorporate training on advanced digital tools, new biomaterials, and personalized treatment approaches to ensure that practitioners are well-equipped to leverage these innovations in their practice.

Ethical considerations will remain a crucial aspect of this evolving landscape. As new technologies and techniques are developed, it will be important to address concerns related to patient privacy, data security, and the equitable distribution of advanced dental care. Ensuring that technological advancements benefit all patients and do not exacerbate existing disparities will be essential for the future of minimally invasive dentistry.

In conclusion, the future of minimally invasive dentistry is set to be marked by remarkable advancements and transformations. The integration of advanced digital technologies, innovations in biomaterials, personalized approaches, and the expansion of tele-dentistry are poised to redefine the landscape of dental care. These developments promise to enhance the precision, effectiveness, and accessibility of minimally invasive treatments, ultimately leading to better patient outcomes and a more proactive approach to oral health. As these trends continue to unfold, dental professionals must remain adaptable and forward-thinking to fully harness the potential of these advancements and shape the future of dental care.

As we anticipate the future of minimally invasive dentistry, it is crucial to consider how evolving technologies and shifting paradigms will reshape practice standards and patient care. The trajectory of this field is increasingly directed toward harnessing the power of innovation to enhance precision, reduce invasiveness, and optimize outcomes.

One of the significant advancements anticipated is the integration of digital workflows into routine practice. Digital dentistry has already begun to transform clinical procedures by offering more accurate diagnostics and treatment planning. Emerging technologies, such as high-resolution intraoral scanners and advanced imaging systems, are set to further refine these capabilities. These tools provide a comprehensive view of the oral environment, enabling practitioners to detect issues at their earliest stages and plan interventions with unprecedented precision. The continued evolution of these technologies, coupled with the integration of artificial intelligence, promises even greater advancements in diagnostic accuracy and treatment customization. AI algorithms will increasingly analyze complex data sets to predict dental issues before they manifest clinically, allowing for more proactive and preventive care.

Advances in biomaterials are another key area poised for significant development. The field has already seen remarkable progress with the introduction of highly durable and aesthetically pleasing materials. Future innovations will likely focus on enhancing the properties of these materials to further mimic natural tooth structures and improve their longevity. The incorporation of nanotechnology in biomaterials is expected to bring about substantial improvements in strength, wear resistance, and even self-healing capabilities. These advancements will enhance the performance of restorations and contribute to more durable and long-lasting results, aligning with the principles of minimally invasive dentistry that emphasize preserving natural tooth structure while achieving optimal functional and aesthetic outcomes.

The concept of personalized medicine is also set to revolutionize minimally invasive dentistry. As our understanding of genetics and individual health profiles expands, personalized approaches to dental care will become more prevalent. Genetic information may provide insights into an individual's susceptibility to various dental conditions, allowing for more tailored preventive measures and treatment plans. This personalized approach aligns with the minimally invasive philosophy by focusing on early intervention and customized care, thereby minimizing the need for more invasive procedures.

Tele-dentistry, though already gaining traction, is expected to further evolve and integrate into mainstream practice. The ability to conduct virtual consultations and monitor patients remotely offers significant advantages, including increased access to care for those in underserved areas. Future developments may see enhanced tele-dentistry platforms that facilitate real-time diagnostics, remote monitoring of treatment progress, and even the provision of certain preventive and therapeutic interventions. This will make dental care more accessible and convenient for patients, aligning with the minimally invasive approach of reducing the need for physical interventions through early and remote management.

Educational frameworks for dental professionals will also need to adapt to these changes. As technological advancements become integral to daily practice, dental education will increasingly incorporate training on new digital tools, advanced biomaterials, and personalized care strategies. Preparing future practitioners to effectively use these technologies will be crucial for the successful integration of these innovations into patient care.

Ethical considerations will remain a vital component as the field progresses. With the expansion of digital and personalized technologies, issues related to data privacy, consent, and equitable access to advanced care must be carefully managed. Ensuring that these innovations benefit all patients and do not exacerbate disparities in dental care will be essential for maintaining trust and promoting equitable healthcare.

In summary, the future of minimally invasive dentistry is poised to be marked by significant technological and methodological advancements. The integration of advanced digital technologies, innovations in biomaterials, and personalized approaches to care are expected to enhance the precision, effectiveness, and accessibility of dental treatments. As these developments unfold, they will not only refine the practice of minimally invasive dentistry but also contribute to a more proactive and patient-centered approach to oral health. Embracing these changes will require dental professionals to stay informed and adaptable, ensuring they can leverage new tools and techniques to provide the highest quality care.

As we explore the trajectory of minimally invasive dentistry, it becomes evident that the future holds the promise of even more refined and patient-centric approaches. The continuing evolution of materials, technology, and methodology will undoubtedly shape how practitioners address dental conditions with minimal disruption and enhanced effectiveness.

The role of technology in minimally invasive dentistry will likely expand, with advancements in imaging and diagnostic tools at the forefront. High-resolution imaging techniques such as optical coherence tomography (OCT) and advanced magnetic resonance imaging (MRI) are expected to become more integrated into dental practice. These technologies offer detailed cross-sectional views of tooth structures and surrounding tissues, facilitating early detection of conditions like carious lesions or structural weaknesses that might not be visible with conventional imaging. The enhanced diagnostic capabilities will support more accurate treatment planning and enable interventions that are both less invasive and more effective.

Another promising development is the increased use of 3D printing technologies. In the realm of dental prosthetics and restorations, 3D printing has already shown considerable potential. As the technology evolves, it will likely enable the creation of highly customized dental appliances with precise fit and function, tailored to the unique anatomical features of each patient. This personalization will enhance the outcomes of minimally invasive procedures by ensuring that restorations and appliances conform more closely to natural tooth structures and individual patient needs.

In addition to technological advancements, there is a growing emphasis on regenerative techniques in minimally invasive dentistry. Stem cell research and tissue engineering are leading to innovative approaches for repairing and regenerating dental tissues. For instance, researchers are investigating ways to stimulate the natural regeneration of dentin or enamel, which could potentially reduce the need for restorative interventions. These regenerative techniques align with the core principles of minimally invasive dentistry by focusing on preserving and enhancing natural dental tissues rather than replacing them.

The integration of machine learning and artificial intelligence (AI) into dental practice is another exciting development. AI-driven systems are already being used to analyze large volumes of dental data, providing insights into treatment outcomes and predictive analytics for various dental conditions. As these systems become more sophisticated, they will assist in the development of personalized treatment plans based on individual patient data, historical treatment responses, and predictive modeling. This level of personalization will not only improve the efficacy of minimally invasive treatments but also contribute to more proactive and preventive care.

The future of minimally invasive dentistry will also see an increased focus on patient education and empowerment. Digital tools such as virtual reality (VR) and augmented reality (AR) are emerging as powerful resources for patient education. By providing immersive simulations of dental procedures and treatment outcomes, these technologies can help patients better understand their options and the benefits of minimally invasive approaches. Enhanced patient education will foster greater engagement and cooperation, leading to improved treatment adherence and overall outcomes.

Additionally, the growing emphasis on holistic and integrated care models will influence the future of minimally invasive dentistry. The integration of oral health with overall health management is becoming more prominent, with an increasing recognition of the links between oral conditions and systemic health. Minimally invasive techniques will be integral to this holistic approach, allowing for the management of dental issues in conjunction with other health conditions through less invasive and more preventive strategies.

Sustainability and environmental considerations are also expected to become more prominent in dental practice. The development of eco-friendly materials and waste-reducing technologies will align with the broader trend toward sustainability in healthcare. Minimally invasive dentistry will benefit from innovations that not only enhance patient care but also reduce the environmental impact of dental procedures and materials.

In summary, the future of minimally invasive dentistry is set to be characterized by technological advancements, innovative materials, and a greater emphasis on personalized and preventive care. The integration of cutting-edge imaging, 3D printing, regenerative techniques, AI, and digital education tools will refine how dental procedures are performed, ultimately enhancing patient outcomes and satisfaction. As these developments unfold, they will reinforce the core principles of minimally invasive dentistry, focusing on preserving natural tooth structure and delivering high-quality care with minimal intervention. Embracing these advancements will require a commitment to ongoing education and adaptation, ensuring that dental professionals can effectively integrate new technologies and methodologies into their practice.

www.ingramcontent.com/pod-product-compliance
Lightning Source LLC
Chambersburg PA
CBHW052137220526
45471CB00004B/1421